Natural and Folk Remedies

CARLSON WADE

Foreword by
H. W. Holderby, M.D.

Parker Publishing Company, Inc.
West Nyack, N. Y.

PRINTED IN THE UNITED STATES OF AMERICA
B&P—13-609990-4

Dedication

To Your Natural and Happy Health

Other books by the author:

Helping Your Health with Enzymes
Magic Minerals: Key to Better Health
The Natural Way to Health Through Controlled Fasting
Carlson Wade's Gourmet Health Foods Cookbook

Foreword

This is a most interesting and fascinating book on natural remedies. The author, Mr. Carlson Wade, is one of today's more brilliant medical writers, and has done a good job of researching this important aspect of natural treatment.

America is a sick nation standing at her drugstore counters trying to buy good health. We stand before the counters like animals before a water trough, thinking perhaps that the drugstore is the spot from whence all health blessings flow, when in reality, many times, the answer to our problems lies in the natural and more simple treatments.

All the rich treasures of the earth and sky have been given us as a free gift. Many of these natural remedies have been used down through the ages successfully in treatment, only to be forgotten as the generations passed. Mr. Wade is attempting to sound an alarm and call us back to some of these good and non-harmful remedies.

We have taken mountains of pills and lakes of liquid medicine in our headlong pursuit of health by the drug route. We are creating a nightmare world of drug-induced diseases. "All drugs are poison"—this is the timely warning of a distinguished physician. He holds, in common with many of his colleagues, that doctors and the public must return to sanity in the use of drugs. Drugs act by interfering with the physiological functioning of the body.

When attacked by disease, many will not take the time and trouble to search out the cause of the illness. Their chief anxiety is to rid themselves of the pain and inconvenience. So instead of taking natural remedies, they resort to patent nostrums, of whose real properties they know little, or apply to a physician for some remedy to counteract the result of their misdoing, but with no thought of making a change in their unhealthful habits. If immediate benefit is not realized, another medicine is tried, then another; thus the evil continues.

People need to be taught that drugs do not cure disease. It is true they sometimes afford a present relief, and the patient appears to recover as the result of their use. This is because Nature has sufficient vital force to expel the poison and correct the condition that caused the disease. Health is recovered in spite of the drug. But in most cases the drug only changes the form and location of the disease. Often the effect of the poison seems to be overcome for a time, but the results remain in the system, and work great harm at some later period.

This book on natural remedies is timely in that we get the treatment for our problems without being harmed by drugs. Let us try for a welcome change, some of Nature's remedies. Nature is God's physician and the gifts of nature constitute the very best of medical treatment, if properly used. We must learn to use these natural gifts that have been placed at our disposal.

These days, if anything is old it is no good, but if it is new it is accepted. Just because a natural remedy happens to be as old as civilization does not mean it is no good or out of date, or any less effective than it was five thousand years ago. So let us not discard some of the older natural treatments that work just as well today as ever.

All of us want to feel better and look better. "Mirror, mirror on the wall, who is the fairest of them all?" seems to be the cry and desire of millions of Americans as well as other world people.

It is my opinion that this book is an important stride in the right direction, on how to stay healthy without the bad effects of medication.

Yours for better health through natural remedies.

—H. W. Holderby, M.D.

A Word from the Author

In my long experience as a researcher, writer, and editor regarding health subjects, I have always been fascinated as to the reported healings accomplished by natural and folk remedies. In my research and travels, I discovered that simple home-made remedies, various folk health practices, and certain natural foods have the ability to help relieve many everyday ailments quickly, and also help improve one's general health. While collecting these secrets of natural and folk healing, I talked with many people who asked me where they could get a book containing natural and folk remedies. This prompted me to organize my collection of these remedies into a single handy volume. Now, I want to share this unusual collection of natural and folk remedies with my readers.

This book has been organized for your quick reference regarding a given health situation, an old-fashioned remedy you may wish to know about, and the many applications of natural and folk health practices. You will note that it offers a wide selection of natural aids for one's well-being, including a dynamic personal appearance, something for every member of the family—a storehouse of health information to consult for everyday use.

The many folk and natural healing secrets and guides in this book have been drawn from various sources, including those of the American Indian, the South Americans, the Europeans, our hardy American pioneers, the mysterious but vigorously healthful Oriental people, and others. One of the underlying benefits of this book is that the natural and folk remedies and procedures reported in it can help you establish a "Nature-Rhythm" defense to cope with daily attacks on your health and well-being.

The various types of natural and folk remedies reported in this book have been effective in the past. They can be equally effective in present-day usage—and, without the use of drugs or expensive medications! It is hoped that you *now* can learn to let Nature help you achieve the daily good health and well-being that you want for yourself.

—Carlson Wade

Table of Contents

    Natural Key to Internal Cleansing—Continued

    OXYGEN: STAFF OF LIFE · *109*
    SUMMARY · *109*

10 How Nature Can Bestow a Healthful Sleep *111*

    HOW TO RELAX YOUR WAY TO RESTFUL SLEEP · *112*
    HOW WATER HELPS PROMOTE SLEEP · *113*
    HOW RELAXED EYES INDUCE RELAXED SLEEP · *114*
    HOW PERSIANS INDUCED PLEASING SLEEP · *115*
    YAWN YOUR WAY TO SLEEP · *116*
    SUMMARY · *116*

11 How the American Indians Used Natural
    Remedies for Strong Eyesight *119*

    THE SIGHT-IMPROVING HERB OF THE SIOUX INDIANS · *120*
    THE HERB THAT STRENGTHENED
        THE EYES OF THE CHEYENNE · *120*
    THE EYE-HEALING SECRET OF THE NEZ PERCÉS · *121*
    THE HERB THAT SOOTHES EYE INFLAMMATION · *121*
    INDIAN-INSPIRED EYE HEALERS · *122*
    WATER: NATURAL EYE WASH · *123*
    HOW EXERCISE CORRECTS VISUAL DISCOMFORTS · *124*
    RELAX YOUR WAY TO SIGHT HEALTH · *125*
    SIGHT-SAVING TIPS · *125*

12 How to Let Nature Rejuvenate Your Glands
    for More Vital Living *127*

    HOW GYPSIES WOULD USE HERBS FOR VIGOR · *128*
    YOGA SECRETS OF IMPROVED GLANDULAR REJUVENATION · *129*
    THE FOOD THAT AWAKENS LAZY GLANDS · *130*
    EARLY BIRD SELF-STARTER TONIC · *131*
    PEPPY POINTS IN CHAPTER 12 · *132*

13 How to Wash Your Bloodstream
    for the Sparkle of a More Youthful Life .. *133*

    HOW EUROPEAN HEALERS USE
        BLOOD WASHING TECHNIQUES · *133*
    HOW HELEN J. RELIEVED HER "TIRED BLOOD" · *135*
    THE FOOD THAT HELPS WASH THE BLOODSTREAM · *135*

1

How Natural and Folk Remedies Can Give You Better Health and Appearance

Take a look at yourself! What would you give or do to be able to roll back the years? How often have you searched for a method, a program, a formula that would turn back the aging clock and restore vibrant youth? Now your hopes may be fulfilled with this book. You hold this book in your hands as the key that may unlock the secret treasure chest of past and present health-bestowing powers.

This book is a compilation of long-forgotten and secretly guarded methods, programs, formulae, kitchen medicines, herbal elixirs, little-known breathing exercises, all drawn from rare books, hidden scrolls, and word-of-mouth "folk" healers. This book will help you ease tension wrinkles, help you revitalize your digestive system and even show you how to feel young again at any age by a long-forgotten method of blood-washing! All of these benefits and many, many more are yours when you draw upon the health and vitality secrets of the past and put them to use right in your own home!

AMAZING SKIN REJUVENATION

One long-forgotten natural healer came to her notice and rejuvenated Mrs. Lillian R., so that she emerged from social withdrawal and looked as radiant and youthful as ever. At age 42, she developed unsightly skin pores, looked much older, had a sallow complexion and was on her way to becoming prematurely old. She worried about her aging skin. She tried the most expensive cosmetics with little improvements. Mrs. Lillian R. became so self-conscious about her aging that she declined public appearances, avoided social functions, and became more and more inhibited. As far as Lillian R. was concerned, her aging skin meant that life was over.

A Little Known Ukranian Beauty Cream Works Miracles

A housemaid noticed her unhappiness and expressed concern. The moody Lillian lamented that she had heard snickers from friends that she was beginning to look her age. She even *felt* old because her skin was sallow and sagging. Lillian told the maid she had tried some of the most expensive lotions on the market, but they did not provide the "face lift" action that she needed. The maid, an emigrant from Ukrania, listened obediently and then said that she herself was over 50—yet her skin was radiant, glowing with pink health, and bubbling over with the flush of youth!

The Ukranian maid said that she looked young and healthy because she followed a folk remedy known to many Balkan peasant women. After a day in the fields, to counteract the effects of the sun, they dab sour cream or yogurt thickly all over their faces. They make a mask of this cream and keep it on for 15 to 20 minutes, until it sinks into the skin. A thin film remains which tightens the pores and helps restore the youthful elasticity of the skin. Then, the women remove the film with warm water.

The magic secret of this ancient but remarkable folk remedy is in the content of lactic acid. This magical ingredient, found in ordinary sour cream or yogurt, is rich in natural and antiseptic microbes which help scrub out wastes and toxics that cause the aging process.

Hearing this, Mrs. Lillian R. scoffed but when she saw that her Ukranian maid (who was ten years older) had such a blooming, beautiful skin, she decided she would try this folk remedy.

For two weeks she used the sour cream mask, applying it thickly to the skin and letting it remain up to a half hour. Then she washed it off with warm water. That was when she noticed her skin texture improving, a pink color returning, an overall youthfulness. This simple folk remedy helped roll back the signs of Lillian's age and she became a happy, healthy social butterfly again.

HOW THIS BOOK PROVIDES BENEFITS-PLUS

The remarkable features of this book make it unique for many reasons. Without leaving your home, without any unusual effort, you can follow these programs and natural healing secrets and enrich your life and health. This book is unusually beneficial for these reasons:

Ancient Health Secrets Now at Your Fingertips

The book is replete with hard-to-find and hitherto inaccessible health secrets from long and forgotten books, manuscripts, scrolls, and journals. It is an accumulation of secrets known to the Egyptians, the Persians, the sturdy American Indians, the energetic Orientals, and the vanished civilizations who left behind fragments of their discoveries of the healing power of Nature. Now, you have all of the most vital secrets of many such civilizations. If you started to search for them yourself, you would spend years and years of looking—it would cost you a fortune in time! Instead, it has all been done for you and is compiled in this treasure chest of secrets.

Natural Health Secrets Can Save You Money

Most of the creams, lotions, ointments, powders, poultices, herbal washes and rinses, as well as the tonics, inhalers, and elixirs, are very inexpensive. If you make them yourself, right in your own kitchen, you can save a tidy sum. Many of the programs outlined are absolutely free of charge—as free as the air you breathe!

Drugless Healing Is Always Beneficial

Many of the methods and programs of the past were drugless; in an era when chemicals and drugs were unknown, ailing persons became healed by means of *drugless remedies!* There were no side effects, no chemical after-reactions, no harsh residue left in the system, no intolerance symptoms caused by the body's resistance to artificial drugs. This book has drawn from many ancient and modern sources of healing and the countless *drugless* remedies will be welcomed by many who seek to ally themselves with Nature.

Folk Healing Is Often
Absolutely Free and Works Speedily

One young man, Philip M., was troubled with headaches as well as recurring "colds in the head." He tried one medication after another and ran up a staggering medical bill. He had an array of decongestants and medical inhalers that would have lasted anyone a lifetime. Indeed, Philip M. would have endured a miserable lifetime, with pounding headaches and colds, had he not been told of a little-known but remarkably effective headache-cold remedy. Most remarkable about this remedy is that *it is absolutely free!* It is based on the Yogi method of breathing exercises. Called *pranayama,* the benefit here is that by following these exercises, you attain conscious control of the normally automatic body function of oxygen flow. These exercises help maintain a steady balance of oxygen and thereby relieve naso-pharynx obstruction. Since choked-off oxygen is the most pronounced symptom of headache-cold distress, the Yogi seeks to free himself from congestion by these exercises.

Philip M. tried these simple and *free* exercises for his recurring headache-cold syndrome:

1. Breathe in through both sides of the nose; and breathe out through one side, closing the other nostril with a finger.

2. Breathe in and out through the same side, closing the other side with a finger.

3. Breathe in through the side that is less blocked, and out through the other side, closing the unused nostril with a finger.

4. If both sides of the nose are so completely blocked that it is either impossible or uncomfortable to breathe in through either side, breathe in through the mouth and out through one side of the nose, as forcibly as necessary. As soon as the one side of the nose opens sufficiently to permit it, breathe in through the open side and stop the mouth breathing. Repeat this set of four breathing exercises for 15 minutes at a time. Continue with one-hour intervals throughout the day. Perseverance is essential to help

oxygenate your system and remove the cause of recurring head-ache-colds.

In Philip M.'s situation, he did these exercises and was able to enjoy a cold-free season. He discarded his medicines. (Occassionally he soon caught more colds because he was careless about keeping his feet warm, about getting proper rest and solid nourishment.) When he allied himself with Nature and lived healthfully, the Yogi *pranayama* breathing exercises became the natural "folk medicine" that helped rid him of colds and headaches.

HEALING OF HERBS

Because the ancients (and even the moderns) were without chemical medicines and drugs, they turned to Nature for healing substances. Herbs have been used throughout recorded history, and probably before. Many of the potions and health elixirs in this book use herbs which are available at most pharmacies for a modest cost. You may also purchase these *medicines from the meadows* from any herbalist. Look in the classified telephone directory of a large city under "Herbs" for possible sources. Keep looking until you find a herbalist who will sell you these healing grasses of Nature. As we shall see, the hundreds and hundreds of herbs that have been used for healing, even during the days of King Solomon, have a treasure of benefits. Herbs can be used for internal as well as external common and uncommon ailments.

How a Herb Poultice
Brought Back Pain Relief

Troubled with shooting pains through her lower back, Clara G., at a youngish 37, decided that arthritis-rheumatism had struck her. She was resigned to her fate. As a saleslady in a large department store, she had to do a lot of bending to reach into showcases. Each time she bent very low, a knife-like pain stabbed deep into her lower back. She cried out from the pain as involuntary tears came down her face. Her "arthritis trouble," as she called it, almost cost her a needed job. She tried remedy after remedy, not to mention some very expensive doctors' treatments. But her painful spasms always returned. What could she do? Accept it?

Clara G. would not grit her jaw and accept the "inevitability" of arthritis distress. She learned that the hardy Vikings used herbs for relieving their forms of arthritis-rheumatism. Since these explorers lived in the damp and cold climate of the North Sea, they were frequently troubled with back and joint distress. Fragments of writings and journals have been unearthed, having been written by seamen and ships' captains who maintained logs of their journeys. It was reported that Eric the Red, the Scandinavian navigator who settled in Iceland as far back as 982, complained of "creaking" of his bones. A year later, when he discovered and colonized Greenland, he brought along with him some kegs of herbs and grasses. These were used to make a poultice as well as an elixir that purportedly relieved his aching joints and restored him to health—and later he became the legendary King of the Vikings.

Eric the Red, as recorded in ship's logs and journals, transferred his herbal knowledge to his son Leif Ericson, who is credited with having discovered North America about 1000 A.D. Young Leif, on his journeys, carried kegs of herbs and nourished himself and his crew. This probably gave them stamina. It is believed they searched for new lands to replenish their herbal supply. After landing at Vineland (later, America), they filled up on herbs and sailed off in good health.

Now, from handed-down writings, we have discovered that the Vikings were remarkably healthy and free from symptoms of backache, arthritis, rheumatism that often plague people in cold climates. Herbs may have been the answer.

Clara G. Takes a Health Tip
from Arthritis-Free Vikings

She read of certain herbs used by the explorers that enabled them to perform rigid ship's work in the dank, damp and foggy climate that often provokes joint distress. She decided to try some.

ARTHRITIS-EASE HERBAL POULTICE   Take one-third part lobelia, two-thirds part slippery elm. (Obtain the herbs in a ground or granulated form.) Mix with water or cornmeal to make a thick paste. Heat. Put over the affected joint and let remain until cool. You may also put the herbal mixture in a little cloth sack, heat up, and then apply to the aching joint. Do not let a poultice become cold. Have a second poultice ready to use imme-diately after removing the first one.

Clara G. experienced relief from this herbal poultice, which she applied to the region of her back where she'd felt sharp pain. She would also use the following folk healer:

HERBAL OINTMENT FOR SELF-MASSAGE   Take equal parts of oil of origanum, oil of lobelia, add a few drops of capsicum or extract of capsicum (red pepper). Mix together. You may apply this full strength or mix with cocoanut oil. Massage thoroughly. Apply directly to the entire affected region and rub gently until the healing heat penetrates the pores and the herbs help relax the spasm.

Why These Herbal Healers Helped Clara

The magic ingredient in these herbs is its powerful *mineral* content. Here we have a nutrient that serves to relax muscles, normalize blood pressure, and cleanse the system of impurities. Herbs are tremendous sources of minerals which help maintain the normal calcium-phosphorus balance so vital to arthritis-free-dom. Clara's aching joints received the benefit of these minerals through the poultice and ointment and this may have been the turning point. Clara's back distress eased and she could soon bend over with scarcely a reaction. She continues to use the herbal remedies at least twice a week to help "mineralize" her aching parts and keep them in a well-lubricated condition. She learned much from the hardy Vikings!

HOW TO STEAM OUT YOUR TOXIC WASTES AND CLEANSE YOUR INTERNAL ORGANS

Palace scribes during the reign of King Nebuchadnezzar of Babylon (604–561 B.C.) report that their revered leader periodi-cally underwent a special "washing" that gave him "the strength of a lion." This famous Babylonian king possessed amazing vital-ity, when we read that he led legions all over the Middle East and personally supervised winning battles. His astonishing mental and physical health could well be attributed to the "washings" that he took once a week.

From various writings about this ancient health restorative, we know that it is the forerunner of today's Turkish bath. This is one of the most remarkably beneficial ways of steaming out your toxic wastes and cleansing your internal organs. It is a folk remedy that provides a self-washing to cleanse your glands and internal organs so they can work without the accumulation of grime, mucus, sludge and waste. Here is how you can self-wash your insides by taking a simple home remedy:

1. Drink plenty of water before and after. Turkish baths produce profuse perspiration which casts off wastes. To avoid dehydration, drink fresh water before you begin.

2. In a closed bathroom, fill the tub with comfortably hot water. *Before* you get into the tub, sit on a stool. Let the temperature (from 105°F. and up) open your pores to enable the sludge-carrying perspiration to pour out. After you have thoroughly perspired, use a rough cloth or hand brush to rub your body thoroughly. Rub away the mucus perspiration from your skin's surface.

3. Now, immerse yourself in the tub for just ten minutes. Take care that the water is *comfortably* hot. Relax yourself.

4. Now, stand up, let the hot water run out of the tub, and use a faucet hose or spray to rinse yourself with comfortably cool water. This will close the pores.

5. Emerging, dry yourself off and lie down in a room where the temperature is about 70°F to 80°F.

Benefits of This
King Nebuchadnezzar Cleansing Bath

By inducing a natural perspiration, you are ridding the body of accumulated wastes and infectious toxic mucus-sludge that may predispose you to illness. This home remedy bath also helps normalize the body temperature, build resistance to colds, ease the nervous system, and replenish the bloodstream, which is often the silt-filled stream of life. It is almost like washing out your bloodstream. Such a self-washing promotes skin tone and color and makes you feel "glad" all over!

NATURE'S TREASURE OF HEALING MEDICINES

By taking advantage of all that Nature has to offer, by using her herbs (medicines from the meadows), her water, her fresh air and soothing sunshine, her abundance of natural foods, her vast secrets of healing, you can help restore, rejuvenate and preserve your precious well-being. This book draws from countless little-known and once-secret records and ancient writings about the power of natural healing energizers.

You will discover how to give yourself a massage and melt aches and pains; you will be amazed at the simple techniques to help revitalize the circulation. You will learn how Nature intended for you to have a soothing and healing sleep without pills! Ever wonder about the superior eyesight and overall health of the American Indian? In this book, you will be taken to the woods and forests of these all-natural people and you will learn how you can rejuvenate yourself through Indian tonics and elixirs.

Easy Exercises for a "Forever Young" Feeling

You will also learn about surprisingly simple stretching exercises, breathing exercises and an amazingly simple walking exercise that can put new life into tired muscles. All this and much, much more await you in the following chapters of this modern compilation of ancient and nearly-forgotten secrets of Nature's healing medicines and tonics. Through Nature, you can look, feel and act younger!

WHAT NATURAL HEALING CAN DO FOR YOU

1. Help restore health balance by using drugless remedies known to the ancients of past civilizations.
2. Save money by following these natural healing programs composed of simple items at modest cost.
3. Drugless healing is usually free of chemical after-effects, harsh residue in the system and distressing side-effects.
4. Nearly all of these natural healing programs can be done right in your own home with no special equipment. Many are absolutely cost-free.
5. Try a sour cream mask for skin beauty.
6. Breathing exercises ease recurring cold-headache problems.
7. Herbs have dynamic mineral absorptive powers to ease joint pains.
8. The Babylonian remedy self-washes and self-cleanses the insides.

2

Beauty Secrets
Using Herbs and Kitchen Remedies

The firm for which Hilda J. worked decided on relocation to another state. Because of family obligations, Hilda J. could not move with them and she started looking for another job in her home city. At age 39, with close to fifteen years of business experience to her credit, she felt confident she could easily find a suitable position. That was when her secure world fell apart.

Hilda J., although a healthy 39, looked much older because of sallow skin, telltale wrinkles, chapped hands, unsightly flaking. She was indirectly told that the vacancy required a much younger woman. This made her all the more upset. That was when she took a good look at her appearance and decided to beautify her skin and make herself much younger. She tried many preparations with average results. Then she tried more natural and so-called old-fashioned beauty tricks and underwent a remarkable transformation. The years of age peeled off and a radiant, charming, *youngish* woman emerged. Now she could meet the competition of youth in the business world. Even though she may have had enviable experience and training, she originally was turned down because she looked old! Appearance is often a decisive factor in success, popularity, social acceptance and romance.

HILDA'S WRINKLE-FREE CREAM   Here is the folklore beauty treatment that Hilda used to help smooth and erase the telltale lines in her face. For a natural facial, mix the white of an egg, herb tea and powdered milk. The herb tea is made by mixing half a

27

handful of rosemary into four ounces of boiling water. Leave to cool for twenty minutes. Strain and store in refrigerator. When this is ready, mix two teaspoons of this herb tea with the white of an egg and one teaspoon of powdered milk. Apply it to the face and leave on for fifteen minutes. Then rinse with cool water. Do this nightly and feel the tightening of your skin muscles and tissues.

BENEFITS OF FOLKLORE BEAUTY BUILDERS

The past and present time-tested home remedies for beauty-building are especially beneficial for these reasons:

Non-Allergic

If you have special chemical allergies or if your skin reacts to standard cosmetics, look to some of the following all-natural beauty preparations that should be non-allergic. Many are made from materials found right in your kitchen.

Minimal Cost

Making these lotions and following these surprisingly simple skin health secrets from the past and present will cost very little. For just a few coins, you can give yourself a beauty rejuvenation every single night. Your budget can always include a natural beauty treatment because of such modest expense.

Grandmother Looked Young with Folk Remedies

Many of the following old-time beauty secrets were used by Grandmother (she made them herself) and she always had peach-bloom cheeks, an enviable rosy glow, and a porcelain cameo beauty that is today considered a rarity. Grandmother looked and felt young with many of these folk remedies which, incidentally, are used in some of our most expensive commercial products of today. Save cost by spending a few moments to make the folk remedies to suit your personal needs.

Beauty Parlor in Your Own Kitchen

Many of these beauty builders can be made right in your kitchen. Just reach into your refrigerator or pantry and mix yourself a beauty treatment. Some of these formulae require items available at most pharmacies for a modest cost. You can have the pharmacist mix them for you and then take home the jars and bottles and give yourself a beauty parlor treatment. Or, you can mix the items yourself. Natural folk and herbal beauty secrets will ease your budget and time problem about going to a beauty parlor.

BEAUTY SECRETS TO REJUVENATE YOUR SKIN

TO HELP CHAPPED SKIN   Prepare a mixture of 4 ounces refined linseed oil, 8 ounces rose water, ¼ ounce tincture of benzoin. Mix together and rub onto chapped skin every night and every morning.

BUTTER FACIAL FOR LINES-ERASING   Mix equal parts of cocoa butter and lanolin (available at any pharmacy). Beat together in a double boiler over hot water; when softened enough, mix smoothly together. Rub in well over the face and neck; let remain overnight and next morning; wash off with cold water. The secret here is that the fat globules of the butter and lanolin will seep into the pores of the skin and nourish the cells that require moisturization to ease lines and wrinkles.

AVOCADO BEAUTY MASQUE   If you want to soften rough, dry skin, make a masque of ordinary avocado pears. Mash the pulp of the avocado and apply it to the dry areas every night for a week. The unsaturated fatty acids in this beauty fruit will stimulate sluggish skin cells to manufacture a healthy supply of sebum (the natural oil that lubricates a youthful looking skin).

LETTUCE JUICE FOR OILY SKIN   Cut up lettuce leaves. Put them in a cheesecloth and squeeze out the juice. Apply the juice on your skin daily to combat the oiliness. The vitamins in lettuce will exert an absorptive action on the excess oil and help drain the film off your skin.

CLEOPATRA'S SECRET BEAUTY BATH   Legend has it that the beauty of the Nile (has there ever been a modern beauty who has such an ageless reputation!) would either slay or banish her beauty slaves after they learned this natural herbal secret. Cleopatra, according to folklore legend, had silky soft and youthful skin (she charmed Mark Anthony even though she was many years his senior) by soaking herself in this herbal bath. Now, you can emulate Cleopatra's beauty secret and be a queen in your own right, if not in your bathtub. Here's how to take a Cleopatra Beauty Bath:

In a cheesecloth bag, place a handful of each of the following herbs: rosemary leaves, thyme, dried mint. Also add a handful of lavender leaves, one peel of orange, one peel of lemon, one tablespoon dried lemon. Toss the tied cheesecloth bag into the tub and pour in very HOT water. Let the mixture steep for ten minutes, then let the bath cool for twenty minutes before getting in. Soak yourself for as long as possible. When you emerge, you'll look and feel refreshed, revived and rejuvenated! (Small wonder that Cleopatra was the beauty of the world!!)

HOMEMADE LIP LOTION   In winter, most people suffer from cracked and peeling lips. Try pampering your lips with this oil treatment to ease wintry elements. Heat some olive oil in a pan. Test on your hand to make sure it is not too hot. Dip a cotton puff into the oil. Squeeze out the excess. Lie down, with oil-soaked puff on lips for 10–15 minutes. The emollient action of the oil will heal and soften cracked lips.

EYE BRIGHTENER   Bathing tired eyes in warm water, to which ½ teaspoon ordinary table salt per pint has been added, will ease fatigue. To relieve puffiness from around the eyes, apply pads wrung out of a solution of one pint hot water and one tablespoon salt. Lie back and relax for a few minutes to let the solution work.

GIVE YOURSELF A SALT GLOW   You will help create a sparkling complexion by massaging your face and throat with a mixture of equal parts baby oil and table salt. The salt friction removes dead surface skin and the baby oil softens emerging skin. Leave the mixture on for five minutes before rinsing it away with warm water. Hand cream may be used in place of baby oil.

FIVE-MINUTE HAND BEAUTIFIER   For red, wrinkled "dishpan" hands, try this natural healing secret from the pioneer days. Those hardy pioneer women relied upon Nature for health and stamina. Soak your hands for five minutes in a basin of warm water to which three tablespoons of salt have been added. The constricting action of the salt will help slough off waste debris and scales and also help soothe irritations. Then rinse and dry off.

MAGIC YOUTH-FACE PEEL   A salesman had to keep up appearances. Good looks and a youthful skin belong to men as well as to the ladies! A man who looks young will feel and act young. This salesman, Louis V., had a good territory but it involved being out in the hot, dusty open. This played havoc with his skin. He did not want to use any creams so was told by a dermatologist that the following natural face peel remedy could work wonders by itself. Louis V. tried it and began to look and feel better. But he neglected using this remedy at least once weekly and his skin sagged so that he looked much older. Now Louis V. has his private face peel wherever he goes. You can try it, yourself. It requires only ONE product that costs very little and is sold at almost all food store outlets.

How to Give Yourself a Magic Youth-Face Peel. First, wash your skin in very warm water. No soap! Next, apply a heavy towel soaked in warm water to your skin for three minutes. Remove. After wringing out a soft linen towel in tepid water containing five tablespoons of apple cider vinegar per cup of water, apply to your skin. Now, cover the vinegar-soaked linen towel with a heavy towel wrung out in very warm water. Let remain for five minutes.

Rub Away Dead Skin Cells. Remove both towels. Rinse your skin in warm water, then take a damp Turkish towel and rub your skin briskly. This last rub is to remove the old, dry skin scales that have been detached and loosened by the apple cider vinegar peel. Your skin will look fresh and youthful and will shine with joyous new life.

Secret of Magic Youth-Face Peel. Simple, ordinary apple cider vinegar is a treasure of the rich mineral potassium. We know that potassium exerts an antiseptic cleansing action in the body and helps fight off bacteria and virus infections. By letting this mineral steep into the skin, you enable the potassium to help tone up the cells and tissues and also wash out age-forming debris. Simple apple cider vinegar can help wash away the years.

Egg Facial Uplift   At least once a week, you should give yourself a raw egg facial uplift treatment. Beat a whole raw egg; if you wish, beat in the juice of one lemon. Apply this as a facial mask over the face and neck. Now lie down and relax for 30 minutes. If you are pressed for time and need to do household tasks, go ahead but—don't talk! Keep your facial muscles relaxed and still for the 30 minutes until the mask has dried and you feel its tightening tingle. Now, wash off the mask with cold water. This egg facial uplift home treatment will help soften lines and smooth out wrinkles. The natural cholesterol content in the egg is rich in ingredients needed to replenish the oil-forming cells and tissues of your skin.

HOME CREAMS FOR WRINKLE-EASERS

A wrinkle is a crease or furrow in the skin caused by changes in the deeper skin layers. In youth, the elasticity of the skin re-shapes it into smooth contours after it has been stretched by a frown or a laugh. But with maturity, the skin loses some of its elasticity. It becomes thinner. Consequently, as a muscle pulls the skin, wrinkles and furrows are formed which do not "iron out" as your expression relaxes. Folds and furrows form at the places of muscle stress.

How These Wrinkle Creams Help Erase Lines

The magic ingredient in the following homemade folk remedies is that of a *fatty* substance. These are fatty creams that you massage gently into the skin and help reduce fine crepe-paper wrinkling. They also help soften the outer horny layer of the skin and get to nourish the lower layer. You may obtain these items at almost any pharmacy. Ask the pharmacist to mix this formula to be assured of a proper blend.

WRINKLE ERASER FOR DRY SKIN   Have a blend prepared of these ingredients: 1½ ounces lanolin, 5 drams petrolatum, 5 drams olive oil, 2 drams castor oil. Apply by rubbing well into the wrinkled portions, every single night. Wash off in morning.

WRINKLE ERASER FOR AVERAGE SKIN   Have a blend pre-pared of these ingredients: ½ dram tincture of benzoin, ½ dram spirits of camphor, ½ dram orangeflower water, 2 drams gelavin, 7 grains powdered alum, 1 ounce glycerine, 4 ounces lanolin. Ap-ply by rubbing well over the skin, every single night. Wash off in morning.

FRECKLE-FADING LOTIONS

Freckles are not merely stains on the outside of the skin; they are irregular collections of pigment in the skin, formed by the pigment cells in an effort to shield the tissues beneath from the sun's rays. In some persons the response to sunlight is a smooth tan, due to an even distribution of these pigment-forming cells.

Why Home Freckle Remedies Are Beneficial

Susan Y., troubled by freckles, was a social wallflower. She became inhibited, introverted, developed nervous tremors. She had many freckles on her face, arms and shoulders. While a pretty girl, she felt that everyone stared at her freckles. She might have developed into a recluse but became a hospital case after having tried a commercial freckle cream that almost burned off her skin! She was told that many freckle creams depend on a strong poison, bichloride of mercury, or ammoniated mercury. This mercury may be absorbed through the skin, causing a poisoning that may damage the kidneys. Freckles are situated deep in the skin and corrosive applications such as mercury, strong enough to remove these spots, may also injure the surrounding skin.

Furthermore, many freckle removers contain salicylic acid, causing a skin peel and bad rash. For this reason, many authorities suggest folk remedies for lightening and fading freckles. Susan tried several of the following after she was released from the hospital. Now, the freckles did fade and she felt she could take her place in the world again. These lotions can be made at home, or you can ask your pharmacist to fill the beauty recipes.

LEMON JUICE LIGHTENER   An old home remedy that helps lighten freckles: Just take lemon juice and splash over freckled portion. Let dry.

FRECKLE FADING LOTION   Mix together these ingredients: 3 drams benzoic acid, 30 drops tincture of benzoin, 1 dram rose water, 5 ounces alcohol. Apply twice daily after washing the face.

FRECKLE-FREE LOTION   Mix together the following ingredients: ½ dram zinc sulphocarbolate, ½ ounce glycerine, 1 ounce alcohol, 2 ounces orangeflower water (U.S.P.), 4½ ounces rose water. Wash your skin with warm water, dry, then apply the Freckle-Free Lotion twice daily.

ACNE AND PIMPLE CREME   Mix together equal parts of pure lanolin, castor oil and glycerine. Melt over mild heat until blended together. Let cool. Put in a glass jar and apply to acne and pimple area. Keep applying daily until the natural fatty content of this home remedy nourishes the skin and causes the necessary astringent action to heal pimples.

ONION POULTICE FOR PIMPLY SKIN HEALING   Old-timers would use this farm remedy: Slice up three peeled onions. Cook the onion slices in shortening until transparent. Let cool. Wrap in cheese cloth and apply to pimples as a poultice. The rich minerals in the onion and the high fatty content work to sterilize the skin infection. Let remain as long as possible.

MINERAL FACE PEEL   Often, stubborn pimples and acne need to be peeled off. One of the minerals, sulphur, is known for creating a natural face peel. Ask your druggist for a product known as *Lotio Alba* or "white lotion." Be sure it is made fresh! Do not buy more than two weeks' supply at once because its rich sulphur content evaporates and weakens on standing. Apply this lotion at night, after washing your face with tincture of green soap. It's great for sloughing off dead and infectious skin cells.

HOW TO BANISH BLACKHEADS

Blackheads are collections of dried, hard, oily material in the oil glands. (*Caution* is the watchword because the imbedded dirt must be removed gently. You may scar or disfigure yourself with sharp instruments or devices. Always seek the aid of a dermatologist, a physician who specializes in skin care, for any chronic skin problem.) Here are several reportedly beneficial home remedies to use for dissolving and easing the blackhead problem.

BLACKHEAD VANISH LOTION   Have your pharmacist mix these ingredients: 1½ ounces stearic acid, 15 drops triethanolamine, 3 ounces distilled water. Nightly, apply this cream to the face after washing with tincture of green soap.

MINERAL-RICH BLACKHEAD LOTION   Have your pharmacist mix these ingredients: 1 dram sulphur, 1 dram glycerine, 1 ounce cold cream. Nightly, apply this special mineral-rich lotion to the face after washing with soap.

OATMEAL FACE WASH   This has been used for more generations than we can remember. It reportedly helps wash away blackheads. Here is the recipe:

    16 ounces powdered oatmeal
     8 ounces powdered almond meal
     4 ounces powdered orris root (at pharmacy)
     1 ounce powdered castile soap

Mix all ingredients thoroughly. Add two tablespoons hot water and make a mash. When of a paste-like consistency, apply to your blackhead area and rub in gently. Let dry and remain one hour. Rinse with cold water. Repeat regularly to wash out the imbedded dirt.

BUSY PERSON'S FACE HEALER   For those of you who are always on the go and need to carry a quick 'n' easy face healing tonic, here's an old-fashioned remedy—ordinary *spirits of camphor*. Buy a small bottle at any pharmacy. Just pat it on any blemish at any convenient and private moment. Keep applying until the blemishes dry up and disappear. You may feel a little "tang," but spirits of camphor helps check infection and also speeds up the healing process. Simple, yet effective!

ICE AWAY THOSE UNSIGHTLY PORES AND BLOTCHES

Ordinary *ice cubes* help to exert a tightening and closing effect on unsightly enlarged pores and blotches. When the oil glands become blocked, the secretion cannot get out and an oily material hardens. The nose and nearby cheeks are most commonly affected. Cold water and ice cubes help cleanse the face and also close the pores. Take an "ice treatment" regularly. Just wrap ice cubes in a cloth bag and apply to the affected region for as long as comfortably possible. This helps diminish overly enlarged and dilated pores.

BUTTERMILK FOR UNSIGHTLY SKIN PORES   The rich calcium and phosphorus content of ordinary buttermilk has a sterilizing effect on the skin. These minerals help reduce overly large skin pores. It was always a popular old-time home treatment. Soak absorbent cotton pads in ordinary buttermilk, pat on your face. Let dry for 15 minutes. Rinse off with cool water. Repeat throughout the day as needed.

SKIN TONE TONIC   For centuries, the famous beauty salons of London and Paris would give their exclusive clients a secret skin tone tonic that helped tighten up the pores and impart a youthful freshness to the skin. (It is believed that Marie Antoinette originally discovered this beauty secret and guarded it jealously until she went to the guillotine. Moments before, she revealed it to her close *confidante*, and thus was created a trend in beauty salons.) After you wash your face, put a few drops of spirits of camphor (sold at most pharmacies) into a basin of water and rinse your face again. Pat dry. The action of the spirits of camphor will tighten up the pores. Small wonder the French Royalists were famed for having such beauties in the Imperial Court of Paris.

HOW FOOD CAN HEAL YOUR SKIN

You may think it odd, but certain fruits and vegetables can actually help your skin heal and "youthify" itself! The magic secret here is in the rich vitamin-mineral-enzyme content of these foods. They work together to create an astringent and soothing effect on the skin. Here are some choice skin foods that you *apply*, rather than eat. (A good idea is to eat lots of fresh fruits and vegetables to help nourish your glandular system which, in turn, nourishes your skin.)

TOMATO MASK   Place a few slices of raw tomatoes on your face and let the juices soak into your skin. Spread mashed tomato pulp over blotchy and affected skin regions.

CUCUMBER JUICE LOTION   Squeeze out the juice of a cucumber, then apply to the skin as you would any lotion. The rich vitamin-mineral supply helps heal infections.

BEAN BEAUTY MASH   Boil fresh green beans. Mash and apply to skin blemishes as a poultice. Let dry and then rinse off in cool water.

ALL-IN-ONE FACE HEALER   Ordinary *cod liver oil* has a healing effect on the skin. If you have acne, freckles, blotches, pimples, rashes, cold sores, sunburn or what-have-you, use ordinary cod liver oil. Just apply liberally and let remain as long as possible before washing off in cool water.

YOUR SPECIAL FACIAL MASSAGE

For maximum skin lubrication benefit, give yourself a special facial massage. The benefits are many. By massaging a cream into your face, you help smooth outlines that are due to moisture loss. You also help cleanse, oil, moisturize and improve skin muscle tone. Massage your face and neck firmly and vigorously with your fingertips; always use *upward* strokes, from your collarbone to your scalp.

PRESSURE MASSAGE FOR SKIN FIRMING   First, contract your face to a definite firmness by smiling—hold it! With a firm pressure and slow circular motion, massage with the *heel of your palms* upward from the collarbone, under and over the chin, moving along the jaws and slowly upward over the front of the cheek, then back and forth over to your ears, and on up over your temples.

The firmer the pressure, the more you will elasticize your tissues without stretching your skin. The benefit may be compared to an ironing process, helping to soften and smooth out deep wrinkles by bringing deep blood circulation into the tissues. Repeat this massage as often as you wish.

HELP YOURSELF TO NATURE'S BEAUTY SHOPPE

A wide variety is available to you from Nature's Beauty Shoppe. Beauty and attractiveness depend upon a well-nourished body, lots of fresh fruits and vegetables, plenty of rest and overall cleanliness. A "natural" beauty is a great rarity. The most attractive person is frequently one who is not bountifully endowed by Nature but who has achieved an illusion of beauty by utilizing poise, good grooming, cleanliness and vibrant, youthful health.

True charm is more than a matter of physical perfection. It is knowing how to use the elements of Nature to help embellish and decorate yourself so you will look naturally attractive and healthfully appealing.

BEAUTY TIPS FROM NATURE'S SALON

1. Folklore beauty recipes worked wonders in a previous age without commercial products.
2. Rejuvenate and refresh by using ordinary food for lotions, creams and face masks.
3. Natural ingredients and reported non-prescription formulae help conditions of freckles, acne, blackheads, wrinkles, pores, blotches.
4. For a modest cost, make skin creams right in your own kitchen, using tomatoes, onions, cucumbers, buttermilk, flour meal.

3

How to Help Nature
Stimulate Rejuvenation of
Hair and Scalp

Leonard B., at a young 33, became alarmed at his progressing hair loss. Whenever he combed and brushed, more hair came out than under average conditions. He also had dandruff. He tried one commercial preparation after another with minimal results. He pictured himself as a balding, oldish man called "Pop" by others who were probably older than himself, but who had hair—the symbol of youth and health. That was when Leonard decided to try some of the old-time healing programs he had heard about.

How Leonard Stimulated Scalp Rejuvenation

He followed instructions outlined in a handwritten manuscript that had been in the family attic, among other heirlooms, for generations. One of his grandparents had written, in a flourishing scroll, that the Indians and the early pioneers had full heads of hair even in advanced age. This grandparent gave a program that was used for those who wanted to have radiant, healthful hair. It was all-natural, too. Leonard began the program:

SCALP RUB   Rub your scalp with equal parts of water and vinegar. Rub vigorously to stimulate hair follicles and to massage the folk lotion into the scalp pores. This helps create an antiseptic action to cleanse out the accumulated toxins and destructive wastes that inhibit hair health.

OIL MASSAGE   Heat ordinary olive oil, a folk healer for hundreds of years, and massage it into the scalp. The rich supply of unsaturated fatty acids in the olive oil help create what is known as an "acid mantle" of the scalp. The skin is normally acid and flourishes healthfully in acid medium.

CASTILE SHAMPOO   Ordinary, pure castile soap shampoo is a mild and soothing way to cleanse the scalp. The ingredients in the castile will soothe itching and also promote favorable scalp health.

DAILY BRUSHING   Use a natural bristle hair brush and do the familiar one-hundred strokes a day. It is suggested that you use natural bristles because the plastic or artificial bristles tend to tear the hair shaft and irritate the scalp.

LEONARD'S HAIR BEGINS TO IMPROVE   After several weeks of following the folk healing program, Leonard's hair health improved. Hair loss abated and dandruff gradually disappeared. His hair soon became healthfully luxuriant and he felt young again! These old-time treatments really work!

HOW FOLK HEALING TREATMENTS
OFFER HOPE FOR YOUR HAIR

An analysis of hair shows it to be composed of oxygen, iron, hydrogen, nitrogen, carbon and sulphur. The old-timers may not have known of this chemical analysis but they knew that certain herbs seem to favor hair and scalp health. Herbs are prime sources of antiseptic ingredients and also exert a toxemia-cleansing action on the pores that determine hair health. In particular, herbs nourish the follicles and papillae, the hair-growing segments of the scalp. Old-time hair health herbal washes are these:

WILLOW TREE HAIR LOTION   From a herbalist or pharmacy, obtain the leaves and bark of the willow tree. Soak in a cup of boiled water (about one tablespoon of the herb to a cup) and when comfortably tepid, soak into the scalp. The rich supply of minerals nourishes the hair shafts to stimulate good scalp health. Use a hair lotion or herbal hair tonic.

HAIR STIMULATING HERBS   Folklore points to the benefits of these herbs (use any *one* of them): nettle, pepper grass, sage, henna leaves, burdock. Steep one tablespoonful in a pint of boiling water for thirty minutes. Massage your scalp with this solution.

Then let dry and comb in the usual way. The magic power of these herbs is in the rich mineral and enzyme action that exert a "come alive" feeling to the scalp.

KITCHEN TONICS FOR HAIR REJUVENATION

To HELP PROMOTE GROWTH OF HAIR   For helping the scalp awaken sluggish follicles, here is a reported scalp pomade to be used the night before shampooing; it helps ease dandruff and has a beneficial stimulating response. Most herbalists or pharmacists can prepare it for you. The following ingredients are to be mixed together and then applied as a pomade: 5 grains pilocarpine hydrochloride, 1 dram distilled water, 3 drams Balsam of Peru, 6 drams precipitated sulphur, $4\frac{1}{2}$ ounces benzoinated lard. Let this pomade remain on the scalp overnight. Shampoo the next morning. The ingredients reportedly help nourish scalp follicles.

For EXTRA HAIR GLOW   After you shampoo your hair, rinse with one part ordinary apple cider vinegar and two parts of water. The nourishing power of potassium will put a thick hair glow into your crowning glory.

To RELIEVE DRY HAIR CONDITION   Shampoo and towel-dry your hair. Then apply a small amount of mayonnaise (about a tablespoon) and leave it on the hair for one hour. Shampoo lightly and rinse. The natural fatty acids help nourish and feed your hair and promote the flow of oil from the sebaceous glands.

For A BETTER HAIRSET   You can add protein and body to your hair by using any vegetable oil (sesame, peanut, castor or olive) as a wave-set. Combine it with small amount of solubilized lanolin such as solubilized isopropyl *or* acetylated lanolin. Apply to your hair; do not rinse out. Let it dry. Your curls will remain for days longer. This is how Grandma had such enviable locks of hair that remained in place for days and days.

To CONTROL OILY HAIR   Dissolve one tablespoon salt in the wave-set lotion. This will control the oily hair and keep it from increasing. The ingredients in the salt will soak up the excess oil and actually "drink" it out of your scalp.

To HELP RESTORE NATURAL GLOW TO YOUR HAIR   Mix one ounce apple cider vinegar and seven ounces of water and use as a rinse after shampooing. This rinse is especially beneficial after permanent waving to give added body to hair. It's called an acidifying rinse because it restores the natural "acid-like" covering on each strand of hair.

To HELP FRIZZY DRY HAIR   Rinse your hair with wheat germ oil, then follow the acidifying rinse offered above. This will help "tame" your hair.

HOW SALT CAN PUT GLOSSY SHINE INTO YOUR HAIR

For glossy, shining hair, try this shampoo: Mix one ounce of orris root (available at most pharmacies) with one-half pound of salt. Rub well into your scalp and then brush out briskly. Your hair will take on body and a natural shine. (Also, you can clean your hairbrushes by rubbing a mixture of equal parts salt and flour thoroughly through the bristles.)

SALT EASES SCALY SCALP   If scaly scalp is a problem, make a pack of one cup salt and five tablespoons water. Make a paste, then rub into your scalp. Let it remain for five minutes. Remove by brisk brushing and then shampoo. This helps rid your scalp of embarrassing flakiness.

HOME SHAMPOOS FOR ITCHING SCALP

A noted physician, who emphasizes old-time healing methods, has found that chemicals in shampoos may often be responsible for and even aggravate itching scalp. He suggests that the hair be cleaned with these folk shampoos for about one month:

EGG SHAMPOO   Beat two or three raw eggs; wet the hair with warm water and rub in the beaten eggs thoroughly with the tips of your fingers. Rinse thoroughly with lukewarm water. Follow with a vinegar rinse, made from one teaspoonful of white vinegar in one quart of lukewarm water. Brush thoroughly while the hair is drying.

SAPONIFIED COCONUT OIL   If you have only a minor degree of scalp itching, you may want to try a special form of liquid soap as a shampoo. Saponified coconut oil, obtained from any pharmacy, is much gentler, more effective and lower in price than most commercial shampoos. It helps nourish the scalp and hair while easing itch, reducing dandruff incidence and promotes a general feeling of good health.

CIDER VINEGAR
AND ITS NATURAL CLEANSING POWER

Dorothy J. thought that women have fewer hair problems than men. At one time, this may have been true because of genetic and hormonal differences; but in our modern times, women are using so many harsh chemical ingredients on their hair, in the form of tints, colors, rinses, permanent waves, bleaching, hair sprays, shampoos and special types of washes, that the hair shafts have become damaged and hair loss is on the increase. Small wonder that when Dorothy began to brush her hair, she noticed several "thin spots" that made her look faded and unattractive.

She gave up her expensive lotions and costly, chemicalized hair cosmetics. Dorothy J. turned to a simple but surprisingly effective folk healer that used just two ingredients. One of the ingredients was absolutely free—water! The second ingredient cast a few coins and was available at any food outlet—apple cider vinegar! Here is what Dorothy J. did to help reduce dandruff and help restore a normal hair growth:

In a basin, put one glass of tepid water and two tablespoons of apple cider vinegar. Daily, moisten your hair and scalp with this solution and use as a natural hair tonic.

PRE-SHAMPOO HAIR TREATMENT   Mix together equal portions of apple cider vinegar and water. Saturate your hair and scalp *before* any shampoo. Leave on for five or ten minutes, then rinse with tepid water. Now shampoo.

Benefits to Dorothy J.

Her scalp itch subsided after a half-dozen such kitchen treatments. Then her hair began to flourish. The benefits of this natural folk healer lie in the highly acid (organic acid) *malic,* plus the life-giving enzymes in the apple cider vinegar. They work together to help destroy the "bottle bacillus," a germ responsible for many scalp and hair conditions; this germ is often responsible for dandruff, falling hair and baldness. Bottle bacilli will clog the hair shafts and impede the production of sebum, a natural oil secreted by the sebaceous glands. The combination of malic acid and enzymes helps detoxify the bottle bacillus and enables nourishment to reach the subcutaneous tissues that are responsible for sending natural oils to the scalp. So we see that, by using this ordinary rinse, Dorothy J. received the benefit of cleansing the follicles and pores that were clogged with bottle bacillus and thereby exerting a nourishing action to the hair. In a few weeks, her hair became lovely and rich and full.

Hair Loss Returns Again

Fully confident, Dorothy J. returned to her array of perfumed hair lotions and tonics. She used so many of these, after getting weekly bleaching at the beauty shoppe, that her dandruff and hair loss returned. Now, the loss was so great, there could be no restoration. Had Dorothy J. adhered to the natural folk healing programs, she might today be sporting natural, lovely hair—instead of a wig!

THE SPANISH HERBAL HAIR TREATMENT

The Spanish men and women have long been known for thick, gleaming, glossy hair. The beautiful and handsome flamenco dancers with their flashing eyes, their shining hair, their trim figures, give a feeling of vibrant youth, even though many are in their late 40's and even late 50's. It is true that your image of youth is determined by the health and abundance of hair.

The Spanish gypsies have several folk healing treatments that have worked, according to reports, to the level that many people will not use any other hair care lotions. For living proof, just look at the thick hair of an average Spanish man or woman. Even the bullfighters who are under nervous strain (often attributed to effect hair loss) have enviable thick and healthy hair. Here is a Spanish herbal hair treatment that appears to have helped their hair beauty.

HERBAL SCALP RUB   Mix one ounce of spirits of rosemary (sold at most herbalists or pharmacies) with one pint of warm water; now mix in the yolk of one egg. Add just a pinch of borax. Rub thoroughly into the scalp. Let remain for five minutes before using the following Spanish Shampoo.

SPANISH SHAMPOO   Slice up one-half pound of pure castile soap. Put in a porcelain pot with two quarts of warm water. Let boil until soap is dissolved. Cool, it should have a thin cream consistency. Now stir in one-quarter pint of ethyl alcohol. Let the mixture soak together (if possible, prepare and let stand for three days in a warm room). Use a small portion as a shampoo. Rinse in cool water.

HOW OIL CAN REJUVENATE HAIR COLOR

The natural emulsion of oil helps to replenish the drying effect of wind, rain, sun, on the hair. Oil further seeps through to the scalp glands and helps to lubricate the shafts.

CASTOR OIL RUB   Rub simple castor oil into your scalp at bedtime. Shampoo the next morning. Begin by doing this twice a week, then go to once every two weeks. The high unsaturated oil content will put life into your tresses and give them a healthful shine. For a rejuvenation-plus effect, try this old-time tip: After you have rubbed in the castor oil, steam it deep into your pores by pressing hot wet towels on the scalp. This enables the soothing oils to penetrate deep within the surface of the scalp.

OLIVE OIL SCALP MASSAGE   Stimulate and rejuvenate your scalp by a simple olive oil massage. Warm ordinary olive oil, then massage into your scalp. For extra benefit, steam in the oils with hot wet towels. Then use a natural shampoo.

FOUR-DAY HAIR RE-GROWTH PROGRAM

Fred McK. was troubled by falling hair. He had tried a variety of past and present treatments, but his hair still fell out to the level where more of it remained on his comb than on his head! At 45, he thought that some hair loss was to be expected, but this was too profuse. It made him so self-conscious that he did not want to go out with his wife and children for fear that he would be mistaken for a grandfather! Fortunately, when he discussed his problem with a herbalist and pharmacist, he was told of a time-tested and rather successful Four-Day Hair Re-Growth Program. Fred decided he would try it. He had nothing to lose except more hair. Here is what Fred did:

On the *first* day, part the hair in small sections and apply white iodine to the scalp with a swab of absorbent cotton.

On the *second* day, part the hair in small sections and massage the scalp with castor oil. Use just enough oil to penetrate the scalp. Too much oil makes a sticky mess.

On the *third* day, repeat the white iodine application.

On the *fourth* day, use a bit more of the castor oil and massage well into the scalp.

Now wring out a very hot towel. Give yourself a steam treatment (be careful not to burn yourself) by wrapping the towel around the head. When cool, remove the towel and dip it into hot water and give yourself another steam treatment. Repeat for four steam treatments. Then let the hair dry and comb and brush the usual way.

FRED'S HAIR BECAME MORE ABUNDANT   This natural folk treatment stopped Fred's falling hair and, where there were thin or shiny spots, a little fuzz appeared. This old-time hair growing program worked for Fred. While in his case it did not restore an adolescent's thick hair growth, it helped him to the point where he felt confident and looked so good that he was no longer introverted and shy. He could go out on the town with his family and not be self-conscious again.

HOW COCONUT OIL HELPS HAIR HEALTH

The rich oil of the coconut is a prime source of powerful hair follicle stimulants. Coconut oil has long been regarded as a magic ingredient to grow hair. Years ago, it was noted that Spanish men who worked at cutting coconut palms, where the oil dripped regularly on their heads, had long, thick and healthy hair.

Coconut oil is available at most food outlets. Just rub and massage it regularly into your scalp to promote hair health. Steam it into your scalp so the precious ingredients dig down deep to nourish the roots of your hair. Coconut oil is beneficial because of its prime content of hair-helping phosphorus and potassium as well as its rich supply of natural unsaturated fatty acids. All serve to lubricate and oil as well as stimulate the function of the hair shaft and follicles. Take a tip from the hair-healthy Spanish and use natural coconut oil as a hair massage and tonic.

HERB TONIC   Stew one pound of rosemary in one quart of water for five hours. Strain. Add one-half pint of bay rum to this tonic. Stir and store in a glass jar. Rub this herb tonic into the roots of your hair night and morning.

PANTRY FOODS FOR HAIR STIMULATION

Many old-fashioned treatments are now the vogue in some of the best hairdressing salons of the country. Ordinary pantry foods are being used for nourishing the hair. These include:

LEMON JUICE   Lemon juice helps bring out natural glow in hair and also is suitable for a natural and mild bleach. The citric acid will also help sponge up excess oil so if you're troubled with oily hair, sprinkle lemon juice with water on your hair and let dry. Then brush and set.

EGG SHAMPOO   The rich silicon and sulphur content of egg, as well as natural fatty acids, helps nourish the hair. Beat an egg yolk with a cup of skim milk. When foam consistency, rub thoroughly into the scalp. Rinse—and keep rinsing with clear warm water until all has been removed. Exceptionally soothing to the scalp. Nourishes the hair, too.

CAMOMILE TEA   Steep one teaspoon of camomile leaves (this is available at most pharmacies or herbalists) in hot water. When comfortably warm, just apply to the hair as a tonic. Let dry, brush and set. It is one of the oldest known means of helping bring out a rich, natural color in the hair.

VINEGAR RINSE   Mix equal parts of apple cider vinegar and water and rinse the hair. Helps make it soft and easy to manage, especially after the hair has been colored.

PROPER EATING TO BUILD
A HEALTHY HEAD OF HAIR AND SCALP

Since your hair requires nourishment as much as all other parts of your body, proper eating will do much for hair stimulation and hair health. Your daily diet should be rich in protein foods such as meat, fish, eggs, cheese, peas, beans, nuts. Obtain valuable blood enriching minerals (the bloodstream carries nutrients to the scalp) from fresh raw fruits and vegetables. Your vitamins are also precious for stimulating growth factors and are available in fresh fruits and vegetables.

Remember to obtain your supply of enzymes, those miracle workers that transform nutrients into the ingredients to help grow hair. Enzymes are plentiful in raw foods which include fruits, vegetables, some nuts, seeds, beans, etc. Proper and healthful food will help give your hair a shine and that all-important elasticity—the quality responsible for bounce, an alive-look and a youth-appeal.

HOW TO BRUSH AND REPLENISH YOUR HAIR

The benefits of brushing include distribution of the oil to the full length of each hair and making it shine; also, brushing is the scalp's exercise that loosens and removes dry dead skin, increases circulation, and removes lint and dirt. Brushing helps stimulate each follicle and makes it come alive and healthy.

Head-Down Position Lets Your Hair Breathe

A daily brushing with a clean natural bristle brush, with your head hanging down, is essential for letting your hear breathe. The head-down position brings blood circulation to the scalp, and makes it easier to use long brush strokes from scalp to hair ends. Brush your hair *away* from your scalp to help revive it, rather than down flat on the head. This aerates your scalp and permits a rush of oxygen-bearing blood to flood and nourish your hair follicles.

HOW MASSAGE CAN AWAKEN SLUGGISH HAIR CELLS

Many people who have pronounced hair loss also have a tight scalp. By loosening up the scalp with this special finger massage, you permit air and a rush of blood to reach the constricted and choked hair cells. If possible, do this 5-minute daily finger massage in the outdoors. If weather does not permit, then open the windows and stand in the middle of the room. A steady flow of fresh air should circulate in the room. Here's how a simple 5-minute daily finger massage can revitalize and restore the health of the hair cells:

1. Take a deep breadth. Hold it, then bend forward from the waist with the knees bent. Push your head as close to the floor as possible. Feel a tremendous flow of oxygenated blood into all parts of the hair and scalp.

2. While in this position, place your fingers on the side of your lower neck and gently push forward. Push up and in front of your ears. While you do this, release your fingers and push your palms above your eyes and across the forehead.

3. Release your hands and your breath as you return to a

standing position. Do this casually. Repeat the massage program five times.

HAIR AND SCALP PEP-UP MASSAGE   Press your hands firmly upon your scalp and move it back and forth, up and down with a circular motion until every portion of the scalp is soft, flexible and moves freely. The skin of the entire scalp should be manipulated. Also beneficial is gentle pinching and kneading. A gentle but firm pulling of the hair improves its strength and stimulates its growth. Pass your closed fingers through every portion of the hair to create an even pulling all over the scalp.

TWO-MINUTE SCALP MASSAGE   A noted doctor offers this suggestion for helping hair and scalp health through massage: "Massage your scalp daily for at least two minutes. Do it this way— hold your fingertips firmly against the sides of your head and move the *scalp itself* with the fingers. Don't just rub the fingers back and forth over the scalp, as this irritates the scalp and breaks off the hairs. Just slowly knead the scalp, going over the entire head in this way. This is beneficial because it increases the blood supply of the hair and is important in scalp care and treatment. Don't scratch or dig your nails into the scalp." Just two minutes per day!

HAIR-RAISING SUGGESTIONS IN SUMMATION

1. Replenish hair health by means of scalp rub, oil massage, castile shampoo and daily brushing.
2. Nourish hair by means of special herbal shampoos and tonics, made right in your own kitchen.
3. Dry, oily, itching and other hair-scalp conditions respond to oil steaming treatments.
4. Wake up a sluggist scalp with simple self-massage for minutes a day.
5. Proper diet and cleanliness through natural shampooing and "head down" brushing help keep scalp and hair in healthful and good condition.

4

How to Wake Up
Your Lazy Circulation
for New Youthfulness

Alice J. was all twisted up when awakening in the morning. Her arms and legs felt like gnarled knots. Each movement was as cumbersome as pushing heavy weights. Alice J. would grimace and bite her lower lip in tension as she clumsily moved her arms and legs to get dressed and prepare for the day ahead. Usually, it took her the better part of an hour before some circulation could be awakened so that her limbs had better flexibility. Even then, it was arduous to do the sweeping, ironing and even the carrying of small bundles. Alice J. scoffed at any chance of relief. She insisted that when a person advances in years, "the circulation slows up and that's it!"

Foolishly, she denied herself the benefits of what is known as *Nature's Circulation Boosters* which exert a revitalization and a reawakening of internal stagnation that leads to "tired blood" even in youth. Alice J. missed out on these natural internal cleansers and surrendered to so-called middle-aged tiredness. When she later developed arthritic tendencies, Alice J. could blame only herself for her impaired circulation.

HOW NATURE'S CIRCULATION BOOSTERS
CAN HELP YOU

Many clinicians and professional healers have succeeded in awakening a lazy circulation and imparting a feeling of renewed youth by means of natural self-friction programs. These natural circulation boosters help pep up the flow of your bloodstream as well as respiratory systems; they help bring the blood to the surface, thus nourishing the miles of arteries and veins that carry precious oxygen to your body systems and glandular sites. They help revitalize sluggish "toxic pockets" which predispose toward arthritic tendencies. Furthermore, these circulation boosters will send a rush of warm and healthy oxygen carrying blood to cold hands and feet, helping to improve their tingling sensation of youthful life.

SELF-ENERGIZER   This Circulation Booster is especially beneficial for an overall body tingle and glow. It helps awaken sluggish cells that may be responsible for that "morning stiffness" we all grimace about. Here's how to give yourself this Self-Energizer:

1. Fill the wash basin with tepid or slightly warm water. (Be sure you have the room warm; in most cases, it could be your bathroom.)

2. From the tepid or slightly warm water, wring almost dry a rough wash cloth. (A regular friction mitt may be obtained at most drugstores.)

3. Rub briskly the left forearm and arm. Rub till the skin is pink. Be sure you continue rubbing until the skin is glowing pink.

4. Dry the arm with a warm towel. That is all for your first day's start on this Self-Energizer.

5. The next day you rub not only the left arm and forearm, but include the right arm and forearm as well. Get the skin pink. The reaction in the skin to the friction and to the stimulating effects of the water does the trick.

6. The third day you rub both right and left arms and add the chest.

7. On the fourth day you rub both arms, the chest, and add the abdomen or trunk.

8. On the fifth day rub arms, chest, trunk and one lower extremity. On the sixth day you include the other lower extremity.

9. On each morning, get the water a little cooler. Soon, you'll adjust to several ice cubes floating around in the basin. For added benefits-plus to give yourself a more vigorous circulation booster,

leave a little more water in the friction mitt or wash cloth. In other words, don't wring it out quite so dry.

10. Should you have a sensation of chilliness, then *dry* each segment of the body before starting to rub the next. Gradually, you should be able to rub the entire body without stopping. This Morning Self-Energizer takes only five minutes and it helps revitalize your internal sluggishness and invigorate the senses to meet the day with youthful enthusiasm.

Benefits of Self-Energizer

What happens when you take this self-friction circulation booster? The blood vessels in the skin are toned up by both the cold and the friction so that they help the heart in the work of pumping blood. You should know that the blood vessels actually can assist the heart by pushing the blood back through the veins to the heart itself. Furthermore, this same treatment causes many blood vessels to open that probably have not been open for some time. This benefits by stimulating an increased circulation and the cold hands and feet are not so noticeable as before.

MIRACLE YOUTH-FACE SECRET   Sagging skin and premature aging is often a symptom of impaired and choked-off circulation. The following circulation booster is directed at the face. It helps increase the circulation, enables the bloodstream to pick up more of the nutrients that are made in the skin when sunshine comes in contact with certain fatty elements. This Miracle Youth-Face helps increase the number of red and white blood cells. The red cells are the ones that carry food to each tissue; they carry away sludge and toxic wastes. The white blood cells are your standing army against infectious disease germs. This Miracle Youth-Face program helps feed your body cells more efficiently by revitalizing the circulation. It's also like giving yourself a beauty treatment right in your own home. Here's how to help tone up sagging face muscles and telltale crinkle lines:

Thoroughly cleanse your face. The best time for the Miracle Youth-Face is in the morning and again at night before retiring. You will need: two large terry washcloths, a drying towel and a bowl of prepared ice cubes beside your washbasin.

Fill the basin with water as steaming hot as you can comfortably endue it on your face. Soak a washcloth in this hot water.

Hold it against your face for one minute. Feel it steam open your skin pores and bring the blood rushing to every cell. Now, soak the other washcloth in ice cold water, or wrap it around several ice cubes. Apply this ice cold pack to your face. Feel it tighten your sagging skin and make you tingle with "aliveness."

Repeat this same hot-and-cold treatment to your neck. After five such Miracle Youth-Face applications, dry thoroughly. It is beneficial to use this home remedy at least twice a day, morning and night, for several weeks. Afterwards, do it in the morning to make your day glow with as much youth as your revitalized circulation.

HOW TO BREATHE AWAY HEADACHE DISTRESS

Arnold B. had problems of stagnation. The symptoms included chronic tiredness as well as recurring headaches. He would feel reactions in his eyesight and have to squint at the daily newspaper. Reading only provoked his eye and head distress. He might have continued on, resigned to his illness, had he not been told of a surprisingly simple and old-time folk healing method of actually breathing away headache distress. It called for inhaling a mixture of ordinary apple cider vinegar and water. It helped ease much of his pounding headaches and gradually he enjoyed improved vision. Arnold B. said goodbye to aspirins and drugs. His circulation was boosted.

BENEFITS OF VAPORIZER   Clogged circulation often has a symptom of pounding headaches, eye distress, sinus congestion, constipation and allergic distress. An accumulation of wastes and toxics impede a natural flow of circulation. The blood cells are choked for air since the bloodstream, the carrier of life's oxygen, cannot reach the sludge and debris that have become locked in body sites. It has been noted that the malic acid, a self-purifying element, contained in ordinary apple cider vinegar, helps loosen up these pocket sites of sludge and even detoxify and cleanse. Headaches are often relieved when this inner congestion is freed.

HOME VAPORIZER FOR HEADACHE RELIEF   In a small pan or basin, put equal portions of apple cider vinegar and water; place on stove and let mixture boil slowly. When the fumes begin to rise from the pan, put a towel over your head. Lean your head over until the fumes are comfortably strong. Now take deep breaths of the cider and water mixture. Inhale for at least 80 breaths. Many have obtained blessed relief in 30 minutes with this home method. The malic acid of the vinegar is thus absorbed in the oxygen and goes to work to create an internal scrubbing that is healthfully healing. This is Nature's answer to headache remedies and pain killers.

HOW TO BATHE YOUR WAY
TO SUPERCHARGED CIRCULATION

Immersing yourself in a special type of bath is helpful for supercharging a sleepy circulation. By letting comfortably warm water open your pores and permitting bath ingredients to soak within and help pep up your circulation, you will be experiencing a wonderful revitalization. Here are the basic suggestions that will benefit your poor circulation:

1. Keep the bath a neutral temperature of about 94°F to 98°F.

2. Soak yourself from 10 to 20 minutes in a well-filled tub that comes up to your neck.

3. After the bath, *pat* your skin dry. Do not rub, since this may cause irritation after the soak. As you shall see, the special natural medications that you put in the bath should *not* be rubbed or rinsed off but left on the skin to help seep into the pores and give you gradual throughout-the-day circulation boosters.

ALKALINE BATH   Add one cup of bicarbonate of soda to a full tub of water. Stir well to dissolve and then soak yourself up to 20 minutes.

STARCH BATHS   Add one cup of ordinary dry starch (a fine, smooth laundry starch) to the water and follow general directions. Benefits include a skin-healing and overall rosy glow to the skin.

COMBINATION BATH   Use one-half cup of dry starch and one-half cup of bicarbonate of soda. Helps exert a zippy and tingly sensation that is Nature's happy response to this stimulation.

OATMEAL BATH   Cook two cups of ordinary oatmeal until well done, place it in a muslin bag and squeeze it into the bath water. Stir regularly so the oatmeal does not settle to the bottom. Immerse yourself thoroughly and let the nutrients of the oatmeal seep through your skin and help nourish and revitalize your circulation.

SALT RUB FOR WARMING COLD HANDS AND FEET

Selma B. was troubled with cold feet in all climates. To add to her problem, she had cold hands. If she had to touch someone or shake hands, it created an embarrassing reaction. (No one likes to hold cold hands!) Poor circulation often sends its initial distress signal in the form of cold extremities. A sluggish and sleepy blood flow cannot reach these distant parts of the body. Selma B. would twist her fingers and toes (even in her woolen socks and heavy duty shoes) and endure her discomfort in abject and pitiful misery. Luckily, when she had a routine physical examination, the condition was brought to light. She was told about a *simple* folk healer that involved ordinary salt. (Aren't most folklore healers just as simple?) She tried it with merciful relief. Gradually, she developed warm and comfortable hands. Here's what Selma B. did:

SALT RUB FOR HAND AND FOOT WARMING   Soak the feet in a warm-water bath to which a cup of ordinary table salt has been added. If especially cold, the feet should be soaked in water as hot as is comfortable. After a 15 minute soak, remove the feet and massage gently with moistened salt to remove dry skin. Rub and rub with the salt to help awaken a sleepy circulation. Then rinse in tepid water and dry thoroughly. Do the same with the hands.

SECRET BENEFIT OF SALT RUB   The coarse granules of the salt create an electrolyte reaction that supercharges a magnetic "pull" and exerts a simultaneous "tug" at the stagnation to help liberate the choked body sites. By repeated friction, these minute "sparks" help revitalize and establish a vital, intracellular, electrolyte pattern to replenish healthful circulation. A stream of warm flowing blood soothes and restores natural tingling to the once-cold hands and feet. Just minutes a day and you can rub yourself to a warm feeling.

HOW TO STEAM YOUR WAY TO SLICK ARTERIES

You are as young as your arteries. It has been reported that in certain parts of the world, such as Finland, the people endure a hardy life even in their 70's and 80's and have surprisingly youthful and flexible arteries. The hardy Finnish people may live in a very cold and arduous climate, yet they enjoy a vigorous feeling of youth long after many of us, who are "old" at forty.

The health secret of the Scandinavians may be in their sauna bath. The benefit here is that the health enthusiast enters the sauna bath (usually in a log hut) which has a nest of rocks under which a fire can be built. The person remains there as the rocks are heated practically red hot. The heat causes a self-loosening and self-flushing of internal debris to come washing out through the pores.

Then, after a few minutes to a half hour of steaming, the person leaves and immerses himself in a pool of cold water. After a few splashes, back in the sauna. Now, a few of these hot-and-cold changes may sound like an heroic regimen to you, but the Scandinavians thrive on it and enjoy a youthful glow and well-lubricated arteries. Apparently, this steaming and then cold water splash helps make the Scandinavians enjoy youthful circulation even up into their nineties. It has long been known that this natural health tonic gives the arteries a well-deserved scrubbing and oiling.

How to Enjoy Benefits of Steam-Oiling of Arteries To simulate the sauna, just remain in the bathroom while the tub is filled with hot water. Do *not* get into the tub, but sit on a stool. Enjoy the benefits of perspiring-out your debris-laden wastes, cleansing your veins and tissue cells. After five to thirty minutes of this steaming, let the hot water run out of the tub. Now, let a cold shower (it should be *comfortably* cold) run freely. Get underneath and rub yourself all over. You will have given yourself a steam-oiling that is similar to the hardy sauna bath.

How This Scandinavian Artery-Washing Benefits Health

The quick change from hot steam to comfortably cold flushes out wastes from the arteries. It first causes dilatation of the arteries and capillaries of the skin to the maximum, seen in the rosy-red color of the skin as fresh blood is brought to the surface. Then the jump into the cold water compresses the arteries thus whisking the blood from the skin surface into the warmer viscera or inner parts of the body.

Helps Revitalize Internal Energy

This to-and-fro flushing of blood steps up the circulation. Its faster rate flushes possible sludge from the arteries, keeping the smooth muscle walls of the arteries soft and elastic instead of allowing them to succumb to hardening and arteriosclerosis tendencies. It is reportedly believed that this quick flushing of blood within the arteries helps clear them of cholesterol and other debris or waste products that accumulate to harden the lifelines of the body.

CONTRAST BATHS FOR BODY STIFFNESS

Minna W. had to give up her knitting, much of her sewing, then she was compelled to telephone orders for groceries. Her "morning stiffness" had progressed to all-day stiffness and she found it painful to bend her wrists, elbows and fingers. She would hold on to the arms of her chair as she struggled to get up. Her knees were stiff and would "creak" with her efforts to get about.

Minna W. might have become an invalid, a victim of joint-stiffness, had she not remembered Grandma's old-time "circulation tonic." It was a hot tub-cold shower tonic that pepped up her body organs and restored a youthful feeling to the circulation. Now Minna could move her fingers and legs and blessed mobility was restored.

THE TONIC BATH   The benefit of this "Grandma" healer (she probably learned it from the Indians) includes its magic jogging of the circulation. It helps invigorate and revitalize your internal system and jog it out of the rut into which middle age has probably directed it. Many who have responded happily to this Tonic Bath are so exuberant about restored vigor that they take it every morning to give them power for the day ahead.

How to Free Stiff Joints with the Tonic Bath. Soak yourself in a comfortably hot tub (104°F.–112°F.) for just fifteen minutes. Stand up. Drain the tub. Start your shower with lukewarm water. Gradually, lower the temperature. Turn around to expose your body to the stream at each stage. When you feel the tingly and exuberant cold range, rub briskly with both hands in the region where the shower stream strikes.

You may gasp a bit at the feel of the cold shower stream. This is a reaction that indicates a freeing of hitherto "locked in" debris that may be responsible for arthritic-like stiffness. You will not actually feel cold because the after-effects of the hot tub help keep warm blood pumping through your skin. This action further serves to wash out the slough that has impeded a free internal flow.

When you feel the least bit cold, stop the shower. Dry off briskly with a Turkish towel. Rub yourself until you feel an internal glow.

Added Benefits of Liberated Circulation

It has been reported that those who take a nightly Tonic Bath, as outlined above, enjoy a feeling of relaxation and "toning up." There is also a general revitalization of youthful energy and vigor. Many have reported that they get less colds, have a more normalized blood pressure, and an enviable young skin glow. Once Nature has helped scrub away the debris-laden veins and washes out the internal sludge, the sparkling goodness radiates in a feeling of "get up and go" and the lazy circulation has awakened to a life that is filled with the joy of health.

VITAL POINTS IN REVIEW

1. Pep up your blood circulation with the Self-Energizer.
2. Help restore youthful qualities with the easy Miracle Youth-Face program done in just minutes in your bathroom.
3. Home vaporizer helps you breathe away headache distress.
4. Supercharge the circulation and awaken to vital living with a natural home healing bath using starch, oatmeal or salt.
5. Salt rub yourself to warm hands and feet.
6. Steam-oil the arteries the way the hardy Scandinavians do, right in your own home.
7. Free stiff joints by boosting circulation with a simple Tonic Bath.

5

Self-Massage:
Time-Tested Folk Secrets
for Melting Aches and Pains

Some 3,000 years ago, the Chinese Mandarins learned that stiffness and aching could be relieved by properly applied rubbing and massage. Throughout the centuries, others have enjoyed a melting of aches and pains by having sore muscles relieved through gentle and soothing massage. Homer, the Greek epic poet-author of the *Iliad* and *Odyssey* back in the 9th Century B.C., also referred to healing massage and pleasant stroking. Hippocrates, the acknowledged Father of Medicine, around 460 B.C. recommended massage for bruises, disorders and health improvement.

In ancient Rome, the wealthy used massage as luxury healing in connection with their baths. The gladiators would strengthen and lubricate their muscles and joints by means of massage. In the Orient, massage became an established and recognized branch of healing. As the benefits spread throughout the world, massage became a profession in the Scandinavian countries, where schools were established for the training of skilled professionals in this healing art. Today, there is hardly a country or city that does not have a trained person to administer massage. The miracle healing power of massage is so phenomenal that many persons have learned how to self-rub, so to speak, and experience a melting of aches and pains. By knowing and understanding the basics of this ancient healing art, you can give yourself a healthful massage.

HOW SELF-MASSAGE CAN BENEFIT YOUR HEALTH

A prominent doctor has observed that the muscle fatigued by work will be restored much quicker and much more thoroughly by massage than by rest of the same duration. While the amount of muscle power after a 5-minute rest is increased to only 20 percent, after a 5-minute massage the increase is as much as a hundred per cent or even more. Self-massage of tired muscles relieves the sensation of fatigue and makes the muscle actually stronger.

Helps Soothe Nerves

Sedation is an important physiological effect of massage. The benefits include muscular relaxation and an easing of mental tension. Slow and superficial skin stroking stimulates the sensory nerve endings and helps create a soothing, relaxing sensation.

Self-Massage
Is Beneficial to Heart Health

Those who stand a great deal (such as salespeople, factory workers and even the average housewife, who does most of her work on her feet) may have an impaired blood circulation. When upright, body gravity may tend to cause an accumulation of blood in the lower extremities, the legs and feet. Self-massage helps the heart get the blood out of the legs and back again, to be repumped. The rubbing and kneading action stimulates muscles and blood circulation, returns stagnant blood to the heart, rids the legs of old blood, and renews the supply with new blood pumped by the heart.

Self-Massage Eases
Problem of Waterlogged Tissues

Lymph fluid, which swells in the tissues to lead to conditions such as edema, is best returned to the heart by normal activity and exercise as well as self-massage. Kneading fingers help move the accumulated water and fluid collection to other parts of the body, relieving waterlogged or swelling tissues. In particular, self-massage has been seen to reduce body fluid collecting in the legs and dependent portions of the body; this is especially beneficial for the heart-concerned person and one who must stand for prolonged periods.

Self-Massage Helps
Melt Arthritic Aches

Creaking and painful joints respond healthfully to self-massage. As you move muscles by self-kneading, you also move joints through their range of motions as well. Because joints have a rather poor blood supply normally and in the aging and arthritic condition, we see how vital to health activity self-massage and full range of motion can be. Self-massage helps stimulate a full range of motion of joints and thereby eases congestive arthritis aches.

Self-Massage Benefits
a Reducing Program

Many who reduce should fit a self-massage program into the slenderizing goal. Self-massage moves fat about and helps reduce fluid within a fatty hip or an overly plump backside. Self-massage has a "secret" benefit of moving wastes and fatty clumps around from one body part to the other. This helps redistribute fat and also helps in the elimination of overweight in combination with a proper diet plan.

Self-Massage
Eases Painful Spasms

As you rub and knead, self-massage actually "milks" lactic acid (a pain and fatigue causing substance) and other abrasive waste products from your muscles, thereby easing painful spasms when you bend over or have to go through average range motions of arms and legs. Much soreness is relieved through self-massage.

Self-Massage Creates
an Overall Tissue Energizing

The unique head-to-toe benefit lies in the double-barrel benefit. In self-massage, it is you who receives the exercise as well as the massage. While you are massaging certain parts of your body, you will also be exercising hands, arms and shoulders, lubricating these muscles and joints, helping to nourish the millions of tissues and cells with a fresh supply of oxygen-carrying blood. It's like awakening your body to renewed health and vigor. The most welcome benefit is that self-massage energizes the tissues by increasing the blood flow to the smaller blood vessels.

Perhaps you have noticed that certain body parts become dull and lifeless because of insufficient activity and sluggish circulation. (Women usually have such sluggishness on the inner part of the thighs and upper arms, as well as the abdomen.) Self-massage will help melt this numb, flabby feeling. Self-massage thus puts youthful feeling into the flesh, helping the entire body become mobilized into healthful vitality.

THREE BASIC SELF-MASSAGE MOTIONS

There are three basic forms of self-massage which you can easily give to yourself:

1. *Stroking.* Vigorous rubbing with the hand, usually in one direction also known professionally as *effleurage*).

2. *Kneading.* Picking up the flesh, tissues and muscles, pinching between the thumb and fingers and squeezing. It includes squeezing, or rolling movements, applied with greater pressure (also known professionally as *pétrissage*).

3. *Rolling.* Moving and vibrating the flesh and muscle around the bone, so that it becomes as flexible and easy as rubber.

Other self-massage motions include:

Pressing, tapping. With your fingertips, you beat a gentle rhythm upon the skin and joint.

Thrusting. Hands and fingers reach into the deeper parts.

Hacking. Gentle striking of the muscles with the inner edge of the hand.

LUBRICATE THE PARTS TO BE MASSAGED   Put several drops of any oil or cream on the palm of one hand and rub over the portion to benefit from self-massage. (*Important:* Since the blood in the skin flows from the extremities of your body toward your heart, *always* make your massage movements toward the heart.) Cover your skin with any oil or lotion to give a love-to-touch feeling. Put just a light film of oil on the part to be massaged.

HOW SELF-MASSAGE EASES LEG STIFFNESS

Benjamin R. thought his legs were stiff because of much stair climbing. But when he winced with muscular tightness while getting up from a chair (sitting down caused such gnarled feelings, he dreaded the needed motion), he became concerned. He applied commercial liniments and found that the act of rubbing in the lotion provided more relaxation than the actual product. That was how Benjamin R. began self-massaging his legs and was able to ease his painful kneecap spasms and stiff joint. Here is a self-massage for the legs:

Start with the stroking motion, going upward from ankle to knee. Press firmly and strongly, slightly cupping the palms. Make the upward stroke heavy, the return downward stroke almost a caress. Begin in front of the flesh of the shin-bone and continue around to the calf, the back of the leg. Continue for five minutes.

After the stroking motion, begin a self-rolling massage. Grip the calf and roll it around the bone. Then work the flesh of the shin back and forth against the bone.

Next, slowly continue on the upper part of the same leg. This constant stroking and self-rolling massage will help accelerate the blood flow and ease congestion of the arteries and other blood vessels of the lower leg. Continue upward onto the thigh.

When you reach the thigh, follow the same sequence of self-massage as on the lower leg—begin with the stroking motion from knee to hip, putting lots of weight and vigor. Then, in the kneading, work strongly on the flesh. Pummel and work it. Twist the sinews, twang the muscles, knead and roll them until your upper leg fairly glows with indignation—and life! Then, repeat the same self-massage with your other leg, first the lower, then the upper portion.

How to Self-Massage Youth into the Hips   After the legs are tingling with life, begin with the hips. Lie on the right side, attack the flesh and muscles of the left hip with both hands, rubbing and working with a circular action, kneading it to the bone, and rolling the flesh over the joint. After five minutes, lie on your left side and do the same self-massage to the right hip.

SELF-MASSAGE POWER INTO THE DIGESTIVE SYSTEM

This self-massage program takes just ten minutes in the morning. It helped Adele T. end her lifelong addiction to laxatives. Adele was often embarrassed by her constipation because she would take one of those "night pills" to make her "regular" in the morning. But she feared going out of the house in the morning until the pill did its work. This made her stay close to home for hours and hours, unable to visit friends or to do her shopping. She tried one laxative after another but, instead of making her "regular," they only made her "irregular" and ailing. She once attended a lecture (in the late evening when she felt safe to venture away from the bathroom) and was told that self-massage of the adbomen is extremely beneficial.

How Self-Massage Can Create Digestive Regularity

Adele T. discovered that stomach massage stimulates the motion of the digestive organs, has a rousing effect upon sluggish liver and bowels (organs of elimination), also releases any pockets of gas that might accumulate. Invigorated circulation is thus restored to tired digestive organs by means of ordinary and drugless self-massage. Adele T. discarded her laxatives, began a 10-minute morning Stomach Stimulating Massage, as described. But when results were slow, she gave them up and returned to her laxatives. Only when she became desperate and this time faithfully followed the program could she enjoy normal and healthful regularity.

STOMACH STIMULATING MASSAGE   Lie on the back. With the heels of the hand, rub the stomach so that you move the whole layer of fatty flesh which lies over the stomach muscles. Let it be the loose tissue that moves, not your hands. Use a circular movement with both hands. Continue for five minutes.

Now, sit upright. Pick up the fatty flesh and work it thoroughly, pressing firmly. Change to a churning up-and-down action to bring new circulation to this stomach area. Rub from side to side over your diaphragm, then up and down. Continue for five minutes.

For Added Benefits: One hour before this Stomach Stimulating Massage and one hour after, drink a glass of freshly prepared fruit juice. This lubricates the digestive system and will help normalize internal functions.

SELF-MASSAGE YOUR CHEST   Begin the stroking massage over the rib cage area of the chest, using your palms on the flesh over the ribs in a simulation of rubbing garments over a washboard. Use circular and up-and-down motions. Seize the flesh and roll and twist gently. Work the entire chest and shoulder area; include the armpits where you knead and twist the flesh. Catch and roll any fatty flesh around the center of your waist and sides. Massage firmly. Just ten minutes per day will help revitalize this region containing your respiratory tract. Those who wish to help their breathing health will benefit from chest massage.

SELF-MASSAGE ENERGY INTO TIRED ARMS   During self-massage, your arms will be stimulated but they should also be given this time-tested energizer. Follow procedure similar to that used on the legs.

SELF-MASSAGE AWAY YOUR NERVOUS TENSION

The ancients were aware of tension at the back of the neck. We know that the royalists of the court of King Louis XIV and Marie Antoinette would employ special healers who would rub and massage the backs of the necks and thereby help ease pounding headaches. Apparently, life in a French Royal Court had its stressful situations. Self-massage helps relieve taut muscular tensions and soothe frazzled nerves.

YOUR TENSION-EZE SELF-MASSAGE   Locate your vertebrae at the base of the skull in the back of the neck. Gently, with your fingertips of both hands, pull or stretch the muscles and cords away from the spine in the neck, on either side alternately. Hold the forehead with one hand, pull and push each vertebrae in turn. Reverse hands and repeat.

Wring your neck by grasping the head, one hand at back of head, other on chin, twist it around as far as possible in all directions. Repeat for a total of five minutes, then rest. The tension should slowly begin to melt away.

HEADACHE MELTING MASSAGE   After you have followed the preceding Tension-Eze Self-Massage, progress to this Headache Melting Massage. Relax your head. Let it lie on one shoulder. Then gently roll it over one shoulder, across the chest, over the other shoulder, then across the back. Repeat several times. Now lie on your back on a table or bed. No pillow or head cushion. Slowly, turn your head from side to side. Repeat several times. Taut muscles and wringing-tight tendons will slowly relax and the impinged blood circulation will flow more easily, relaxing tight tension-causing head pains.

HOW TO MASSAGE AWAY BACK STIFFNESS

Young Barry D. worked at a draftsman's table most of the day. No doubt, his hunched up faulty posture was responsible for his recurring back stiffness and backache. When he straightened up after such a position, he would wince with shooting spasms of pain. He lost many working days because he was frequently doubled over with such back pain, he could scarcely get out of bed in the morning. When he was given postural advice by the company doctor, his distress was eased, but he still had recurring episodes of back pain. He scoffed at massage, saying it was just a rubdown and would do him little good. His co-workers enjoyed back flexibility because they followed good postural pointers and also helped their stiff muscles with self-massage. Barry D. was satisfied with partial recovery. This could have led to complete back health if he would have followed simple time-tested self-massaging of the back.

How Self-Massage Promotes Mighty Atlas Back Strength

Legend tells us that the mighty Atlas (the Greek titan who supported the world on his shoulders) would strengthen his back by means of self-massage. With good health, the following Mighty Atlas Back Strengthener should invigorate the shoulders and back and ease taut muscles.

The secret of this special self-massage is in the firm pressure that expands the capillaries (the tiny thread-like blood vessels) and speeds up drainage of pain-aggravating fluid. This, in turn, stimulates cell metabolism, eliminates wastes and increases lymphatic and venous circulation. In that way, the healing of back distress is aided by the following Mighty Atlas Back Strengthener.

BACK STRENGTHENER   Make a fist of one hand. Lying face down, reach behind and press the knuckles of this fist against the near side of your spine. Reach other hand around from other side of back. Grasp wrist and assist pressure by pulling. Select a vertebra and exert this double press and pull on it. Go up and down the spine on one side. Reverse positions of hands and repeat. Instead of reaching around with the helping hand, reach across your chest, place hand on opposite shoulder and assist by shoving. Both positions are efficient. Use the one you are best suited to.

THE MILLION DOLLAR ROLL   Here is a simple motion
that helps relieve tension of the spinal column and thereby restore
free-flowing circulation. Much tension is caused by tightness of
these portions. Professionals call it the "Million Dollar Roll"
because of its value. Lie on your side with upper leg forward and
over the under leg; place hand of under arm on other shoulder;
place hand of upper arm on back of hip of upper leg. Now shove
in opposite directions with each hand. This particular self-massage
helps loosen up an aching joint. Repeat several times.

SELF-MASSAGE FOR GREATER FINGER FLEXIBILITY

Gloria V. developed such stiff fingers and wrists that she could
scarcely write a letter or hold a fork without a grimace and sensation of a shooting spasm. She fearfully envisioned herself a help-
less invalid. She remembered her parents succumbing to
rheumatoid arthritis and confined to wheelchairs in abject pity
and pain. Gloria V. was on the verge of collapse thinking of such
a fate for herself. And she was still in the prime of her life! She
could not endure having her husband and children wait on her
like an invalid.

Of the many healing methods she tried, massage promoted
general well-being and partial restoration of joint flexibility.
She could not afford weekly trips to a licensed masseur, but she
could ask one for a home program. He gave her a self-massage program that helped ease the stiffness and, with a program of professional treatment, stemmed the tide of rheumatic distress. Now
Gloria V. could face life with flexible courage. Here is the
program:

Fingers—Grasp each finger in turn and while holding with
your hand, stroke and knead from tip to base with your thumb.

Back-of-hand—Grasp hand firmly, then work and knead
between bones with thumb.

Massage arm—Begin with: *ROLL*—Raise your arm straight
up in the air. With your other hand, roll the muscle on the bone.
WRING—Twist the flesh of the arm as far as you can without
slipping, then quickly release it. This method is improved when
you let go quicker than the flesh can spring back. *BEAT*—Make
a fist of your hand and beat the entire arm but do not touch bones
or hand. *HACK*—Strike the arm rapidly with the side of your

little finger. If the fingers are extended (open) just as you strike, then the ring finger hits the little finger, the middle finger hits the ring finger and the first finger in turn hits the middle finger. Try it. Gentle "hacking" helps free sludge in the circulatory system. *SLAP*—Slap the arm with the palm of the hand.

(*Note:* The five preceding self-massage motions are done once to the arm. Work your hand fast but cover ground slowly enough to do a thorough self-massage. Don't leave gaps between your hits!)

VIBRATE—Grasp the hand, shake the arm in little quick rhythmic ripples, a sort of shivering, quivering, too-fast-to-see movement. FINISH: Repeat the lubrication movement but this time *without* a lubricant. It is the last soothing, caressing touch.

BEAUTY WITH SELF-MASSAGE

A beautician uses the technique by an upward rub or stroke and a roll between the thumb and fingers. Massage to nerve site may be applied at a notch in the jawbone an inch or so back from the point of the chin. Also, near the back angle of either side of the face, under the cheek bone, at temples and above eyes on bone of brow. Self-massage helps keep skin pores healthy and increases the action of the excretory glands, actually helping your skin to cleanse itself. Self-massage arouses tissues, perks up every little cell, creates a tingling of well-being. With self-massage, the oxidizing power of the blood helps you burn away fatty spots. The accelerated blood flow will tune up the flesh, help consume waste tissues and make you feel and look youthful.

MASSAGE VITALITY INTO YOUR SCALP   Many people who tried this HairGro Massage have told me they actually experienced invigorated scalp health. It requires just several moments and is beneficial for scalp vitality. *Here's how:* Start at the hairline, massage with fingertips gently over whole head, pressure down the back of head. Massage over temples, pressure to sides of head and down neck. Massage over top and sides of head will help bring blood to the hair roots. Stimulation helps loosen tight, dried skin on head. Blood nourishment exerts improvement over scalp skin and hair.

HAPPY NERVE MASSAGE   Because most nervous disorders stem from tensions and headaches, massage should be directed at relieving head pains. For your Happy Nerve Massage, straighten out the curve of your neck by stretching the back of your head toward the ceiling. Simultaneously, push your chin back and down as if you are trying to tuck it under your head. Remind yourself continually of this new way of balancing your head for a few days and it soon becomes automatic. This is a "no hands" type of massage and your neck muscles actually give themselves a loosening up! The benefit of this Happy Nerve Massage is a relaxation of strained neck muscles on the roots of nerves which lead to the scalp area. Soothe and relax these nerves and you have happy nerves!

HIGHLIGHTS OF HEALING SELF-MASSAGE

1. Gentle self-massage is of benefit to heart health, eases water-logged tissues, soothes arthritic symptoms, benefits a reducing program and exerts a youthful energizing effect upon the mind and body.
2. The three basic self-massage motions, stroking, kneading, rolling, can help provide body exhilaration and improved well-being.
3. Before self-massage, apply light oil film to enable hands to slide easily over body. Rubbing a dry body can cause skin irritation by tearing and breaking off the hair.
4. Ease leg, hip and arm stiffness with self-massage. Correct digestive disorders with proper massage and diet health.
5. Relax tensions, back stiffness, scalp tightness with self-massage,
6. How to give yourself a Happy Nerve Massage.

6

Easy Steps for
Happy Feet and Youthful Legs

Janice F. manages a busy household, carries heavy bags of groceries with youthful agility, walks miles and miles in her home as she does the laundry, house cleaning, kitchen work, picking up after others, telephone and doorbell answering. Yet Janice F. is alert on her "happy feet" because she has taken a tip from handed-down natural healers. She has been able to revitalize her foot and leg reflexes by means of several simple home self-energizers. These "happy feet" energizers reportedly eased leg cramps and helped invigorate overall function. Here is what Janice F. does to revitalize foot power:

"CURL TOE" LIMBERING FOR LEGS   Stand with the feet flat on the floor. Curl the toes under. The folks who reportedly used this leg-limbering exercise would do this "curl toe" exercise a number of times whenever they had tired feet. The benefit here is that this "curl toe" forces the arches up and sends a flush of oxygen bearing power through the entire foot, thereby energizing its function.

TIPPY-TOE LEG STRENGTHENING   Old-timers would dance the quadrille for hours on end and show little signs of fatigue. Their secret was this folk exercise: Stand with feet flat on the floor. Slowly, rise as far as comfortably possible on tiptoe. Then lower the feet to the floor. Repeat. This is more beneficiary if done at frequent intervals throughout the day. Grandma would do it whenever she had the slightest feeling of foot tiredness.

LEG RAISING FOR GRAVITY PULL   Here's an oldie that

Janice F. liked to try whenever she felt tired, in general. Generations ago, they realized that this particular motion *reversed the gravity pull* and sent a flush of nourishing blood throughout the lower body, helping to re-stimulate sluggish portions. Janice would lie flat on a couch or bed. She would put several cushions beneath her legs so that they would be a line higher than her head. She would recline in this "gravity pull" for about thirty minutes, then arise as refreshed as could be. Of course, many modern beauty salons have discovered this health secret from the past and offer "beauty boards" to their leg-tired patrons. The benefit is the same with cushions. Janice F. managed her busy schedule with these home healing secrets by using cushions.

SECRETS OF FOOT REFLEXOLOGY

It has been reported that as far back as the days of the Crusades, foot-weary marchers and leg-exhausted pilgrims, who walked over rough terrain for hours at a time, would become miraculously rejuvenated by means of an ancient technique known as *foot reflexology*. This same home practice has been used with complimentary praise in modern massage parlors and foot health salons. It is believed to have originated in the region of ancient Persia and flourished in the comfort-loving age of the Baghdad of Harun al-Rashid and Scheherazade. The soft carpets and deep rugs of the palaces apparently were not without their foot-fatiguing problems. Royalists maintained special foot reflexologists who were trained by the old masters to recognize the vital nerve-zone pressure points of the feet. By proper self-manipulation, the zones could be activated to send rushing streams of nourishing oxygen and vital elements to invigorate tired and aching legs. The time-tested healing method of foot reflexology is slowly gaining prominence in our modern but still foot-weary generation.

Health Secrets of Foot Reflexology

By pressing the fingertips into the soles and heels of the feet and by exerting a mild but deep-compression action on tired nerves, a natural type of healing response takes place. This self-massage helps create an acceleration of blood circulation through tired portions, thus pepping up vitality and endurance. Thus, when circulation is stimulated, body vitality increases and there is an overall refreshment. The ancients would have their private foot reflexologists perform this rejuvenation for just ten minutes per day. Small wonder that pilgrims and Crusaders could cover thousands of miles with "happy feet."

THUMB PRESSURE FOR INVIGORATED FEET   The ancient foot reflexologists would sit in a hard-backed chair. They would take their own feet, one at a time, and apply a thumb pressure to exert an overall rejuvenation. The reflexology was given with a slow rotary motion, using a firm pressure with the flat of the thumb, beginning with the portion beneath the toes, going slowly to the "ball" under the big toe, then to the center, and gradually working downward to the arch instep. Gradually, they would use both thumbs and exert a series of gentle but firm pressures on the entire underside of the foot. Afterwards, they would repeat the same process with the other foot.

Reflexology Helps Relieve Clogged Nerves

The benefits derived here include the dissolution of accumulated crystals clogging nerves and tissues; constant firm but gentle thumb pressure comes in contact with the crystals at the nerve endings that cause obstruction and circulation impairment. By freeing the nerve endings from the clogged crystals, which are dissolved and carried away, the strength and health of the feet become invigorated. Just a few minutes per day helps improve the entire foot and leg health by means of reflexology.

Reflexology Relieves Stagnation

One young man was embarrassed and also frightened by the appearance of clogged veins on his legs. Arthur W. had heard of varicose veins but never thought he would develop them. When he spoke to others, he was told it was "just one of those things," and to accept it. He looked to Nature and foot reflexology. He learned that stagnation often leads to congestion in the legs; circulation is cut off and blood accumulates in veins and arteries predisposed toward varicose veins. He tried several foot reflexology motions, this time using both hands to exert a gentle but firm pinching-kneading compression on the entire leg. He would begin with the ankle, then press fingertips up and down the leg, pulling the calf muscle to one side, then the other, going up to the knee cap.

Arthur W. would repeat this same deep compression home

healer with the other leg. He would do this several times a day. (It is especially beneficial in the morning after the legs have been "asleep" all night and needed stimulation.) He also did it at night to help stimulate leg circulation. After considerable time, the bulging eased up. But Arthur W. erred in believing that one quickie healer would do the trick and that he could continue abusing leg health by faulty posture and poor general body care. His varicosities remained, in a lesser condition, and he resigned himself to his fate.

Foot reflexology is one "oldie" healer that benefits—*if performed in conjunction with overall body and leg care.*

SIX WAYS TO PUT LIFE INTO YOUR LEGS

Invigorate your feet and enjoy improved health by these easy-to-follow, leg-energizing steps to fitness:

1. Walk around tiptoe in your bare feet and stretch up. You'll remember to do this one regularly if you pick out a regular trip; from wash basin to bed at night, for example.

2. Again in bare feet, try picking up marbles or a pencil with your toes. This helps exercise your toes, as well as limber up your arch.

3. Sit down with your feet on the floor, pointing straight ahead of you. Curl your toes under and then, heels still on the floor, turn your feet toward one other. Hold for a count of two; relax for a count of two. Repeat ten times.

4. Walk alternately on the inner and outer edges of your feet, keeping soles off the floor as much as possible.

5. After bathing, stand on the end of the bath towel and try to "rake" in the rest of it with your toes.

6. Just too busy to think about exercises? Then don a pair of exercizer sandals (sold at most footwear and natural food store outlets) to wear shopping or around the house. A special metatarsal crest forces the toes into a gripping position in order to keep the sandals on, and at the same time, flexes the arch. These sandals provide especially good exercise for feet that have been wearing high heels for a full day.

WALK YOUR WAY TO FOOT HEALTH

You've been walking for years, but did you know that the WAY you walk and stand can affect the structure of your feet?

What's more, when you walk and stand correctly, chances are you'll have more get-up-and-go than the person with a sloppy stride. Here are ways to walk your way to improved foot health:

Keep Toe Straight. In walking, keep your toes straight ahead. As you take each step and put your foot down, weight should come down on the heel and then the ball of your foot.

Walking Rhythm. Try to develop a walking rhythm, with springy steps, and then go at it with a steady, easy pace. When walking on an upgrade or upstairs, take two short breaths, then forcefully exhale. You'll have less premature fatigue.

Standing Without Strain. Point one foot (it doesn't matter which one) toward the person to whom you're talking. Bring the other foot behind it at a 45-degree angle, with the heel of the foot in front against the instep of the one in back. Weight should be on the ball of the back foot.

EASING FOOT CRAMPS   Here's a little trick that may be restful if you must stand for a long period of time: roll your feet over, so that you stand on their outer borders with the soles facing each other. This helps melt foot cramps.

FOLKLORE HEALERS FOR FOOT DISTRESS

Old-fashioned folklore healers relied basically upon country store supplies. Today, these are available in most pharmacies and major supply outlets. You may mix them yourself or ask the druggist to do it for you.

FOOT PERSPIRATION   Mix one ounce powdered orris root, three ounces of zinc oxide and six ounces of ordinary talcum. Shake this powder into your shoes or rub onto your feet. Reportedly helps absorb excessive perspiration.

Corns and Calluses

These often result from the effort of the toe to protect itself from irritation. Pressure of the shoe causes a knotty thickening of the skin with the formation of a central core. This hard center in turn presses on nerves beneath and causes pain. Folk healing treatments relied upon home lotions, as follows:

CALLUS SOFTENER   Mix together 15 grains potassium hydroxide, 4 drams glycerine, 2 drams alcohol, 2 ounces distilled water. (Your pharmacist can prepare this home healer for you.) Apply nightly until the callus is soft enough to be removed. For a persistent situation, apply 5% salicylic acid in collodion solution (prepared by your druggist) to the region for three or four days; reportedly, the callus should then be peeled off.

CORN REMOVAL   Take a hot foot bath, then apply the preceding 5% salicylic acid in collodion solution to the corn; repeat application morning and night for four days. Then, soak the feet in hot water again; the corn usually loosens and can be easily lifted out. Apply alcohol as an antiseptic. The corn should come off *easily*. Never force it out. If it is stubborn, continue the applications for several more days.

BUNION-EASE PAD   A bunion is an inflammation of the joint at the base of the big toe. Generally, bunions are caused by pointed shoes which crowd the big toe over and press too much on the joint. A bunion pad often brings relief and gives the painful inflammation a chance to subside.

SPECIAL SHOES FOR BUNION RELIEF   It is reported that bunions will be relieved by wearing a pair of low-heeled lacing oxfords for everyday wear. Have your shoemaker attach an anterior heel, which is a block of leather toward the front of the arch which spreads your weight to the foot bones instead of letting it roll up on the ball of your foot with each stride.

CONTRAST BATHS FOR
STIMULATING FOOT CIRCULATION

The old-fashioned water healer helps stimulate and regenerate foot circulation. Fill a basin with moderately hot water (105°F) and then fill another with moderately cold water (50°F). Soak the tired feet in the hot water for five minutes, then in the cold for only *one* minute; now go back into the hot for another five minutes. Continue for thirty minutes. Always begin and end with the hot water. Then dry off and apply talcum powder. The old-timers would restore youth to their tired legs with this simple water healer.

Foot Bath-Massage Program

We see old portraits and sketches of tired travellers resting beside a stream; they soak their weary, aching and downright miserable feet in the fresh flowing waters, then give a self-massage that stimulates the legs and puts joy back into walking. These time-tested folksy foot healers can still help tired feet and make them happy feet.

FOOT BATH   Sit on the rim of a bathtub. Turn on the water faucet to make a strong flow. Alternate comfortably hot and comfortably cold sprays. Let your feet be revitalized by first a hot flow, then a cold flow. Do this for just five minutes. Always begin and end with a hot flow. You may obtain a convenient spray attachment, that is easier to manipulate, from your druggist.

FOOT MASSAGE   Tired travellers would first soak their feet, then self-massage after drying. All moisture had to be dried off. Modernists sprinkle baby powder over the feet to provide even more relaxation. Massage the soles of the feet in a rotary motion; then massage the sides and ankles in the same rotary motion. Exert plenty of comfortable pressure. (The ancients realized that the more pressure, the more vigorous the compression healing, and the more circulation was sent into the feet.) This also helps "milk" out the toxic material wastes from the feet and improve circulation. After five or ten minutes of foot massage, lie down with upraised feet to further facilitate circulation and maintain healthful body gravity. Rest for a half hour.

SIMPLE FOOT SOAK   Mix together 2½ drams borax and 1½ ounces of sodium carbonate. Dissolve in a basin of comfortably hot water. Soak the feet for thirty minutes.

Hillbilly Foot Duster

In the mountainous and rocky regions of the Tennessee hills, folks often soothe tired feet with these homemade healers:

MORNING FOOT DUSTER   Mix together 2½ drams borax and 2 ounces ordinary talcum powder. Just sprinkle on the feet in the morning to give yourself a peppy start for the day.

FOOT-EASE POWDER   Mountain folk who complain of tired, aching feet, look to "hillbilly lore" for relief. Mix togther: 3 ounces fuller's earth, 3 drams boric acid, 2 ounces store-bought talcum. Shake over tired feet. Rub into feet, too. Folks in the country areas can get these ingredients from the country store. City folks can have a druggist prepare the powder. Helps pavement-tired feet as well as mountain-tired feet.

Foot Scrubbing for That "Leg Tingle" Feeling

A department store clerk told me that she follows this easy 3-step foot scrubbing program that makes her legs tingle with glad-to-be-alive reaction. Bernice W. at a youngish 56, is able to stand on her feet for hours at a time because of proper care. Here is Bernice's own 3-step Happy Feet Program:

1. *Scrub Job.* With a handbrush of moderately stiff bristles, scrub the feet with ordinary soap and warm water. Go all over the feet, soles and heels included.

2. *Toothbrush Treatment.* Use a worn-out toothbrush soaked in soapy warm water to scrub at those inaccessible places. Go all over to help cleanse the accumulated grime and debris. Then rinse your feet.

3. *Pumice Stone.* Rub an ordinary pumice stone on any part of the foot that feels tough. Use a gentle, rotary motion over the heel, the balls of your feet. This helps to soften the skin and discourage callus and corn formation. Then dry and fluff with talcum powder.

Sounds simple but Bernice W., who stands on her feet all day, regards it as her "Happy Feet" Program. She wouldn't be without it.

CREAM AWAY ROUGH SKIN　　Ordinary castor oil that is rubbed into rough and chapped skin on the feet will help create a softening and smoothening action. Rub in the castor oil; let it soak in. Then wipe off with a washcloth and apply talcum or antiseptic powder which is helpfully drying.

ROLLING PIN EXERCISES FOR ACHING FEET　　You may use an ordinary rolling pin. You might want the new kind with designs for cookie rolling which help stimulate the nerves of the feet. Here are two reportedly strengthening exercises:

1. While seated, roll the pin on the floor from tip of toes to heel. Put all the pressure you can take on the right foot and the left foot at the same time.

2. Stand straight. Roll the pin from toes to heel, putting as much possible pressure with one foot, then the other. This simple Rolling Pin Exercise reportedly benefits by stimulating the nerves, tendons and muscles of the lower extremities.

SOUTH SEA FOOT HEALTH SECRET　　You may have marvelled

at the superior health of the people of Hawaii. They have reportedly enjoyed absolute foot health. Why? The secret is simple. These Hawaiians walk barefooted in the soft sand and soft turf. For many generations, many have spent lifetimes this way and have marvelously healthy feet. Of course, modern folks cannot go barefooted all the time, but an occasional or regular barefoot exercise is helpful.

Walk on a clean lawn or sand for at least 30 to 60 minutes (or more) daily. *Secret benefits:* Walking on sand acts as a stimulant to all foot tissues; the sand fits the contours of the sole and arch, acting as a stimulator at the same time. The small sand grains invigorate the skin by a naturally abrasive action.

Take a tip from the healthy South Sea islanders and walk in sand to help revitalize and invigorate tired feet.

SUNSHINE HELPS FOOT HEALTH   In a Swiss sanatorium, persons with aching or ailing feet are given localized "feet sunbaths." The benefit here is that the feet alone are exposed to the fresh sunshine for regulated doses per day. The feet thus absorb the rich supplies of the sun which helps stimulate the function of specific glands beneath the surface of the skin. The oil glands secrete Vitamin D that helps nourish the bones and circulatory system of the feet and legs. Localized or controlled "feet sunbaths" are an ancient healing program for the feet.

LOTION FOR PERSPIRING FEET   Before the days of glamour lotions for perspiring feet, folks would prepare a mixture of the following: 1 ounce eau de cologne, 2 drams formalin, 2 ounces distilled water. Mix together and apply this lotion to the perspiring feet, every night for a week. Or, sponge the feet with grain alcohol every night and every morning.

LOTION-PLUS FOR PERSPIRING FEET   Reportedly, this home "feet brew" offers something extra to help ease offensive odors of perspiring feet. Mix together, or have the druggist prepare: 1½ drams vinegar, 1½ ounces alcohol, 1½ ounces cologne water. Sponge the feet with this lotion every single night, for a week.

YOUR FEET: FOUNDATION OF HEALTH

The foot is Nature's engineering marvel. Your feet contain 52 bones (one-fourth of all the bones in your body), 114 ligaments and 38 muscles. In your lifetime, you will walk more than 70,000 miles or almost three times around the world. On a very few inches, you balance and carry a load weighing more than a hundred pounds and ranging up to six feet high, or more. And depending upon your occupation, you may spend as much as three-fourths of your waking hours on your feet. So keep them in good condition and they'll serve you well as your foundation of health.

TIPS FOR HAPPY FEET IN THIS CHAPTER

1. Refresh your feet with helpful "Curl Toe" and other reported beneficial exercises.
2. Foot reflexology, a time-honored and ancient healing method that is being discovered today. Easy to self-compress your feet in a matter of moments for healthful stimulation.
3. Nine easy-to-follow leg-energizing steps help lead to fitness.
4. Corns and calluses, foot perspiration, bunions, tiredness, find relief through folk healing programs.
5. Scrub, cream and "rolling pin" helps put new life into old feet. Sunshine, a natural foot-warmer, is a Swiss secret that can be enjoyed anywhere the sun shines. Foot happy Hawaiians serve as inspiration for "sand walking" away your foot cares.

7

Time-Tested Folk Applications
for Relief of Backache

By improving your back, you are rewarded with related health benefits. It has been reported that backaches often lead to faulty postures that prompt a bulging abdomen, bent neck with recurring headaches, nervous tension, and a feeling of stiffness in the upper shoulders and back of the neck. A healthy back provides benefits such as a "light feeling" of the shoulders, a clear mental attitude, youthful figure contour, firm muscles, improved digestion. A young-feeling back is a young-feeling body!

Sedentary Causes of Backache

One specialist, who treated countless patients for low back pain, reported the following: "The big muscle groups used in managing the body in various positions and movements are rarely used adequately by the sedentary person. The abdominal muscles are kept slack; the back muscles, while used to keep the body erect, are used in a static rather than dynamic fashion.

"The muscles of the lower extremities are not given any strengthening exercises at all and are usually held in positions producing shortening of the hamstrings. It is this static and unbalanced use of the body which plays an important role in the etiology of the increasingly frequent low back pain."

Furthermore, lack of exercise has led to more backache cases than during the "pre-car" and "pre-lazy" days. A key to easing backache is in more movement and exercise.

MORNING BACK EASE EXERCISES

Following a night of sleep, the spinal column may become a bit stiff from remaining in a fixed position. Here are five very simple back-loosening exercises that take moments per day and help provide release from back tensions:

1. LEG RAISING   Stretch out on your back, flat on the bed or on the floor. Raise your right leg from your hip until it is at a right angle with your body. Slowly lower it to level position. Do the same with your left leg. Do this Leg Raising five times in succession with each leg. Keep the toes pointed and the leg rigid. Between leg changes, rest and relax. Gradually, increase to 10 motions. The reported benefit here is to provide mobility to your legs and hip.

2. DOUBLE LEG RAISING   Lie flat on your back. Now, raise both legs at once. Keep them close together, stiff. Your toes are pointed. Raise to a right angle. Bring forward toward your head as much as is comfortably possible. Now lower slowly to flat position. Repeat five times. Slowly increase to 10 times. Do not strain yourself. If you feel tired, then stop and rest. The benefit of the Double Leg Raising is to help tone up the muscles of your hips and provide greater youthful flexibility.

3. INTERNAL FITNESS TONIC   Stand up. Slowly, as your body below the waist remains *rigid*, bend your trunk sideways; first to the right, then to the left. Your waist is like a hinge. Bend in each direction as far as possible. Raise your hands up to your armpits in rhythm with this Internal Fitness Tonic, simulating the motion of hand pumping a tire. This should be done five times, then increased to ten times. This is a time-tested exercise Tonic that helps "squeeze" the insides and thereby stimulate sluggish organs. Many health clubs and backache healers suggest such a natural "tonic."

4. ARM SWING   Stand up. Breathe in deeply and expand your chest. Whirl your arms in a circle from your shoulder, duplicating a windmill. Begin by making a circle from front to back, then repeat with the contrary motion. This particular Morning Back Ease Exercise helps loosen up tight arm joints and also provides a greater flexibility to the spinal column.

5. NECK ROLL   Much backache distress stems from a feel-

ing of tightness in the nape of the neck. Many old-timers who would hunch over a table and feel a stiffness, would do this surprisingly simple Neck Roll for great relief. Stand straight, but comfortable. Let your head hang heavily forward. Muster up the power of your neck muscles. Roll your head to the right, back, left, then forward. Repeat 5 times. Then rest for several moments. Next, repeat the Neck Roll in the opposite direction: left, back, right and forward. Also, repeat 5 times. For greater neck mobility and tension-ease, make your head heavy so it will help stretch and loosen up your neck muscles. Many have been rewarded with a smooth, youthful neckline in addition to relief from back pain through this Neck Roll.

THE BACK TENSION-MELTING PROGRAM THAT HELPED FRANCES V.

The attractive, youngish Frances V. complained that her back was giving her so much trouble, it felt like it was actually "caving in." Added to this distress were the related pains in her legs. Often Frances would sob out in pain as a knife-like spasm tore through her lower back when she tried to bend over and pick something up from the floor. She was thoroughly examined, yet nothing organically wrong appeared on charts. Frances V. wailed that the agonizing pain was getting worse all the time. Something had to be done.

Prolonged Tension Is Clue to Natural Healing

While Frances V. observed proper bending and lifting positions, she still developed back pains. A clue to the cause was in prolonged tension. With a household to manage, a part-time job, and community social activities and several financial problems, no wonder she was tensed up! This provided a clue to seek natural healing. Tension will make muscles tight and short; if a back muscle is tight beyond a certain point, it starts to hurt like a backache. When Frances stooped, she felt a slight attack. This left the back muscles stiffer and weakened, readying her for the next pain sequence to compound the pain. She sought help from a specialist who suggested these Back Tension-Melting Motions that brought blessed relief:

TENSION LOOSENING   Loosen up your tight back muscles

by wobbling the neck, shoulders, arms, thighs, legs and feet. Lift your arms up slowly, then let them drop. This is an overall tension loosening that takes just 10 minutes.

SHOULDER RELAXANT   Turn the head all the way to the left, then return it to the normal front and center and relax. Now turn it to the right and return. Helps "milk" out tension-causing lactic acid from kinked up shoulder muscles.

KNEE FLEXING   Lie flat on your back with the knees flexed. Slowly draw the right knee up as close as possible to the chest. Slowly straighten the leg, let it fall on the floor limp and relaxed. Put it up again to the flexed starting position. Now do the same thing with the other leg and alternate legs until signs of tiredness appear.

BACK RELAXANT   Lie on the left side; place a pillow under your head so you rest comfortably and your neck can relax. The trick here is to put motion on your back. Now, keep both knees flat and slightly flexed. Slide your right knee as close to your head as it is comfortably possible and then slowly extend the leg until it is completely straight. Let the leg drop to the floor relaxed. Do this three times on one side, then turn over and do the other leg.

Benefits to Back and Mind

The loosening up benefited Frances' back and also helped ease her mental tensions. With a reduced activity schedule and more rest periods, she was able to enjoy freedom from back distress. The Back Tension-Melting Program had provided merciful relief from back spasms. Now she could bend over in comparative comfort. She continues these simple exercises at least one time a week as "insurance" against recurring back distress.

HOW SPINAL-ROLLING OFFERS CONGESTION-FREE HEALTH

The ancients were well aware of the importance of the spinal column for back health as well as for overall fitness. Many specialists have revealed that a well-lubricated and flexible spine rewards the body with healthful organic activities, bodily energies, increased capacity for mental work, better breathing and sleeping, improved appetites and alertness. A flexible spine benefits by offering relief from the susceptibility to digestive congestion, sluggishness, back-muscular tightness. "Look to the spine for healing" has been urged by healers for hundreds of centuries. It offers the "backbone," so to speak, to better health!

How Spinal-Rolling Helped a Mechanic

Anthony R. was in such bad condition, he thought he would have to give up his lucrative mechanic's job. Medical tests revealed no diseased organic conditions. Yet, Anthony R. had to fight back involuntary tears if he twisted at the waist or squirmed in a seat; he had severe muscular spasms that "cemented" his spine in a twisted position. He thought surely he would have to be operated on. Yet, following tests, there did not appear to be any noticeable organic defects. He needed help desperately!

He heard from a fellow-worker, who had once wrenched his back, that "Spinal-Rolling" had helped many others. The fellow-worker, unfortunately, was impatient with his own progress, and while he tried some of the time-tested and natural programs, he could not endure the discomfort. He submitted to surgery and the outcome left him with a permanent limp.

But Anthony R. was willing to be patient and try Spinal-Rolling, and he experienced blessed relief. It took a number of months before some of the pains eased from his spinal column and back distress began to melt soothingly. Here are the five Spinal-Rolling exercises:

1. Lie face down on the floor. Raise to an arched position in which you rest on hands and toes with the back highly arched. Your pelvis is higher than your head. Keep knees and elbows stiff. Drop pelvis almost to the floor but keep elbows stiff; this is vital to help give a "roll" to the spine. As you lower your back, move your head back. Raise it sharply as you lower the body. Take your time while doing this exercise. Repeat a number of times.

2. Lie face down on the floor. Rest on your hands and toes. Arch your back. Raise up slightly and swing the pelvis from one side to the other. Do it slowly and help s-t-r-e-t-c-h your cramped spinal column. Repeat several times.

3. Sit on the floor. Lift up pelvis by putting hands at sides; draw in the feet a little bit. You are now resting on the flat of your hands and feet and your pelvis is just off the floor. Lift up your body. Let your spine be horizontal as you finish the upward movement. Go down to starting position. Go up and down several times.

4. Lie flat on the floor, hands at sides. Bring knees to chest position. Clasp arms several inches below knees. Now pull knees and thighs tightly against chest. Simultaneously, raise your head and try to touch your chin to your knees. Hold this "squeezing" position about ten seconds. *Special Benefits:* Reportedly, this Spinal-Rolling motion sends a wave of energy to the spinal curve where nerves influence the abdomen. It helps stretch and lengthen the spine from tip to tip. This helps overall improvement because stretching of the entire column helps restore a balanced health.

5. Lie face down on the floor. Now, lift yourself up on your palms and toes with your back highly arched. Keep pelvis higher than head. Keep knees and elbows stiff. Walk around the room in this all-fours position.

SECRET OF VERTEBRAE VIGOR

Folk healers of past and present would emphasize Spinal-Rolling because it offered an especial benefit to the vertebrae, the key to better health. Modern anatomical specialists have learned that there are benefits to be derived from simple exercises such as Spinal-Rolling which enabled all the tiny vertebrae comprising the spinal column to separate; this permits Nature to build up the cushiony growths of cartilage between each pair of vertebrae.

Healthful Cartilage for Youthful Spine

The restoration of cartilage helps accomplish a youthful and health-building spinal column, regardless of one's age. Cartilage is a firm but gummy material that gives a rubbery smoothness to spinal movement. Nature does, to a degree, replace the cartilage lost by normal bodily activities which stretch the spine daily. But there is rarely sufficient stretch of the spinal column, in routine activities, to separate the vertebrae in a satisfactory amount. Thus, proper Spinal-Rolling helps keep the back youthfully lubricated and rewards one with a youthful spine.

Nature Keeps Pets in Spine Health

Take a tip from the dog or cat and almost all domesticated animals. The average dog or cat knows about Spinal-Rolling.

Notice how it arches its back, spreads its vertebrae. Have you watched a dog at times lower the front of his body, forepaws extended far before his head and shoulders, writhing and twisting? Small wonder that a dog has such vital energy over so long a portion of his life. Take a tip from the family pet and roll your spine to strengthen the back and overall health.

A FIVE-STEP PROGRAM FOR A YOUTHFUL BACK

Dancers, who are on their feet far more than ordinary, are known for taking time to keep their backs young and flexible. By maintaining foot agility, they maintain their youth by time-tested and traditional exercises designed to "energize" the feet. Many of the royal ballet and dancing academies of the world, for many centuries and right up to present time, insist upon decongestant-exercises such as the following:

No. 1. Stand with feet parallel. Rise up to the toes, then slowly sink down again. Do this about 10 times.

No. 2. While seated, try picking up ordinary marbles with your toes. Pick them up and then let them drop. The benefit here is that this motion strengthens the long tendons attached to the toes.

No. 3. Stand barefooted on a thick, wide book so that the toes overlap the edge of the book. Move the toes over the edge of the book and grip. Repeat several times. Helps strengthen the legs and back.

No. 4. Sit down. Place a pencil betwixt your toes and try to write a letter! This exercise is most beneficial to the entire lower structure of the body.

No. 5. Sit down. Hold your foot with one hand; with your other hand, take your big toe and rotate it around firmly, first in one direction and then the other. Repeat several times. This promotes a "lubrication" of the joints and provides slippery-smooth body flexibility.

HOMEMADE HERBAL POULTICES

Rural and mountain healers of past, and even present, had to rely upon homemade herbal poultices when physicians were unavailable. Many found herbs to be *medicines from the meadows* that could provide the most revitalizing relief to aching joints and distressed backs. Based upon folklore-healing through herbs, here is one such mountain remedy that helped these folks:

HERBAL POULTICE FOR BACK PAIN   Take two tablespoons mullein, three tablespoons granulated slippery elm bark, one tablespoon lobelia, a small teaspoon cayenne. Mix thoroughly together. Now mix with enough boiling water to make a stiff paste. Spread this herbal paste on a cloth. Cover the affected aching portion with the poultice and let remain overnight, if possible. Reportedly helps heal swollen feeling of back and joint pain.

HERBAL LINIMENT   The mountain folk have relied upon a healing liniment that city folk can take advantage of. Take equal parts of oil of origanum, oil of lobelia; add a few drops of oil of capsicum (or extract of capsicum which is red pepper). Apply full strength over aching portion and massage thoroughly.

HERBAL TEA   To soothe tired or frazzled nerves and to help provide internal balm to an aching system, this herbal tea was prepared and used by many of our pioneering predecessors. Mix equal portions of gentian, scullcap, valerian, buckthorn bark. Mix thoroughly together. Use a heaping teaspoon to a cup of boiling water. Take a tablespoon every hour. Increase dose if needed. These herbs are prime sources of natural healing properties that soothe the nerves and help relax tensions. Perhaps our pioneers did backbreaking work, but they had youthful backs and herbs may have been the secret. Our modern folk have every convenience and rarely lift anything heavier than this book, yet yearly, some 28 million hobble into doctors' offices with complaints of back trouble.

Artery-Washing Exercise

Severe leg and thigh pains almost crippled Barry V. While he did a certain amount of walking as a salesman, he also spent much time behind a desk. He was often so doubled over with low-back distress that he could scarcely get up from a chair when sitting for an hour or so. Because he refused to believe that "silly" exercises could relieve his back, he let his condition worsen until he required hospitalization.

Here is one reported Artery-Washing Exercise that is of great benefit by helping to flush out the accumulation of chemical wastes in the leg, thigh and back muscles.

Take time out every two hours when you are on your feet. Remove shoes and hosiery. Lie on your back. Your hips are raised on a pillow. Put feet high in the air. Jiggle them rapidly—but keep your ankles and toes completely relaxed. The secret here is to put full "muscle-milking" power on the feet. Do this for two minutes. Repeat throughout the day as often as possible. This helps wash away the sludge and waste that have accumulated to and in the arteries of the lower body, leading to stagnation and possible back distress. It's your back and your lifeline of health! Look to Nature for spinal mobility and be rewarded with effervescent youth.

SUMMARY OF BACK-HEALING BENEFITS

1. How to wake up and greet the day with a flexible back with the Morning Back Ease Exercise in just minutes, in the morning.
2. Benefits from the Back Tension-Melting Program.
3. Ancient healing of Spinal-Rolling method that lubricates the vertebrae and provides youthful power to the back.
4. A 5-step program for a youthful back.
5. Homemade, all-natural herbal poultices, herbal liniments as well as herbal teas offer a well-rounded folk healing plan for back strength.
6. For probems of leg and low back pain that may be related to varicosities, look to the Artery-Washing Program.

8

The Healing Effects of
Folk Water Remedies

Water has been used from time immemorial for healing purposes. The books of the oldest medical authors make numerous references to the healing effects of water. Hippocrates, the Father of Medicine, back around 500 B.C. extolled the benefits of water application for the healing of many health problems. The ancient Persians and Greeks erected stately and magnificent public buildings devoted to bathing. The Romans surpassed all other nations in the magnificence of their bathing facilities.

Water Heals Illnesses

Two ancient Latin physicians, Celus and Galen, some two thousand years ago, glorified water bathing as being invaluable. Galen maintained that proper bathing as well as applied friction could be regarded as medicine. Others of later years helped revive patients who were fever-stricken, infected, or internally upset with various bathing programs. During time of epidemics and pestilences, the baths were considered a safe refuge from the ravages of infectious diseases.

Vapor Baths Create Self-Cleansing

During the 1600's, public vapor baths flourished in Europe. Ailing patients were steamed and bathed back to health. The self-cleansing action helped scrub out the insides, wash the mucus-covered system, and restore it to sparking clean good health.

Water Healing Gains Prominence

In 1723, a health book entitled *Curiosities of Common Water* referred to water as an "excellent remedy which will perform cures with very little trouble and without charge; it may be truly styled a universal remedy." The noted Victor Priesnitz of Germany, in the 1850's, gained prominence for being a water-healing practitioner. He reportedly cured patients after doctors pronounced them incurable. He even healed his own condition of broken ribs by means of water applications.

This knowledge spread to America, where it was found that the native Indians used water healing as far back as was known. They would emphasize contrast baths for the healing of stiffness, swollen joints and a variety of other common ailments.

The Kneipp Water Healing Program

Father Sebastian Kneipp gained fame by healing Archduke Joseph of Austria, in 1892, of a near-fatal illness, Bright's disease (a kidney inflammation accompanied by albumin in the urine and swelling of body tissues). This helped establish water as a natural healing power to be used in conjunction with general body hygiene. Today, many reports have been made about the healing benefits of water. However, water is not a specific; it is one of the most valuable of many excellent healers. With proper rest, natural and simple food, controlled sunlight, healthful exercise, the body is given the raw materials with which to start a program of self-healing.

True, there are some specific healers for some specific conditions, but not one, and one alone, for all ailments. Several healing sources must be combined to suit the conditions, and not one used to the exclusion of all others. Father Kneipp and others reported on failures of water healing when the person continued to abuse his body through overwork, poor food, lack of exercise and looked to water healing as a sole method. The entire body must be given the benefits of natural invigoration for overall healing.

How Water Healing
Can Be Helpfully Healing

Reports have been made about water healing used to correct conditions of clogged arteries, digestive disturbances, stiff, aching and swollen joints, nerve distress, glandular irregularity, internal organ malfunctioning, allergic tendency, premature aging, loss of vitality, lack of energy. When water healing is used together with the health restorative programs of proper food, rest, exercise, then the benefits accrue.

HOW WATER KEEPS THE ARTERIES ELASTIC

Ronald T. became distressed over his feeling of "tightness" in his arms and legs. Although he was not yet in his 50's, he was told that he had a high cholesterol count and that he would develop arteriosclerosis as well as related conditions of arthritis. Ronald T. loved fatty and rich foods, declined exercise, and looked for an "easy" way to wash his arteries and keep them elastic. He followed a program of self-washing through water. Here is Ronald's program:

For 15 minutes, he would remain in his bathroom while the shower poured out hot water, building up clouds of steam. After letting his pores open up and the steam create an artery-scrubbing sensation, he would then change the shower to brisk cold. He would then hop beneath, run his hands over his body, and, after a few moments, come out and dry himself thoroughly.

Benefits of Self-Washing

The reported benefits of this hot-cold artery scrubbing program lie in the reaction of the water on the circulatory system. The steam opens and dilates skin blood vessels, sending a fresh supply of blood rushing to the surface, then whisking through the body in an effort to create cooling.

The contrast cold causes constriction of the blood vessels; this leads to a quick flushing of fat, cholesterol and waste through the liver and kidneys for rapid elimination. Thus, this program may well dilate, constrict and flush cholesterol from the body, and in the process burn it by elevation of temperature.

Entire Healing Program Is Required

When this inside-washing program is used several times a week, and when corrective and natural foods as well as proper exercise and rest fill a healing objective, benefits are the reward. But in Ronald T.'s situation, even though his arteries felt elastic and youthful again, he still succumbed to a serious decline in health because he ate fatty-laden foods, kept late hours, hardly exercised. There is no compromise with Nature for healing.

HOW WATER SELF-STIMULATES ENERGY

A leading natural healer has reported on a Hot Tub–Cold Shower Program that can actually "jog" your circulation out of the "rut into which middle-age has probably directed it." It is said that this Hot Tub–Cold Shower Program is so stimulating, it is of special benefit in the morning to give you a get-up-and-go feeling. Here's how to do it:

HOT TUB–COLD SHOWER ENERGIZER   For 15 minutes, soak in a fairly hot tub (104°F–112°F). Then stand up, open the tub drain, start your shower with lukewarm water. Slowly, lower the temperature, turning to expose all body parts to the stream. As you get into the cold range, rub briskly with both hands where the shower stream strikes. You may gasp a bit, but you will not feel actual cold, as long as the after-effects of the hot tub keep warm blood pumping through your skin. When you begin to feel the least bit cold, stop the shower. Dry briskly with a Turkish towel.

This natural water healer helps build resistance to wintry temperatures and tones up the circulation, providing alertness and energy. It is further reported that a "feeling of youthful energy and vigor almost always develops after taking these baths regularly, and many patients report that they get less colds, have lower blood pressure, and find a healthier glow to their skin."

HOW A MOIST ABDOMINAL WRAPAROUND
HELPS ESTABLISH DIGESTIVE YOUTH

Betty C. had an embarrassing problem of constipation; in addition to feeling bloated and bilious, she was so "stuffed up" that she felt cramps throughout the night. Added to her digestive distress was chronic sleeplessness. She was determined not to fall victim to the laxative habit. She knew about water healing and tried a simple but effective Wraparound that helped restore digestive regularity, induced a healthful sleep and made her feel "glad all over." This historic natural healer has been used by many people in all parts of the world. It is most popular these days.

MOIST WRAPAROUND FOR DIGESTIVE YOUTH   Wring a strip

of muslin (about twelve inches wide and long enough to go twice around the abdomen) reasonably dry out of cold water. Wrap it around the middle; lap the excess length over so that it is double thickness across the tummy. Fold a heavy woolen strip (twenty-eight inches wide and the same length as the muslin) lengthwise so it is about fourteen inches wide. Wrap it around over the moist muslin cloth in the same manner; it should double across the middle. Pin securely with safety pins. Make sure that all of the wet muslin is covered by the dry woolen; be sure it is tight enough so that air cannot get it.

A tingling sensation is felt. After a few moments, the digestive system should begin to tingle with soothing, relaxing warmth. It should remain overnight for maximum reported benefits. The tingling sensation is a symptom of increased circulation of blood to the middle, thereby easing congestion and bloating. After removing the Wraparound, sponge the body lightly with cool water and rub briskly with a coarse towel. If this is worn nightly, the circulation is given a natural revitalization while you sleep! You'll awaken with digestive tone-up and general improvement.

(*Note:* If the Wraparound is still wet after eight hours of sleeping, you may have used too much water. Or, if the Wraparound gets hot and dry before one gets to sleep, then it was not wet enough to begin with. Make these adjustments and apply before retiring for maximum benefits.)

HOW TO USE HEALING WATER FOR SKIN HEALTH

Many maintain that water will wash away some of the natural body oils. To a certain extent, this has been noted. But water at the same time stimulates the production of more body oil. If you want to combine healing water with an emollient to create skin health, take a tip from a time-honored folk secret: rub lanolin or any vegetable oil into your skin twice daily. This also helps guard against excessive dryness.

OIL THE SKIN FOR BABY FRESHNESS   Noted celebrities have enviably glossy skin. It is reported that a daily soft soak in the tub will keep the skin soft right through summer's drying sun and surf. Rub ordinary baby oil over the body, right down to the toes. Now loaf in a tub of tepid water up to thirty minutes. Then rinse off; use a fluffy terry towel to rub your skin to gleaming satiny beauty. Just the sheerest film of baby oil will cling to your skin to give it a velvety look and help reduce moisture loss.

Salt Rub Away Your Tensions

Ralph J., a much-harried attorney is subjected to increasing tensions. He relieves much by a healing method known back to the days of ancient Babylon. Ralph soaks himself in a warm bath for just ten minutes. He then massages his skin with dry salt. He does this vigorously, from his shoulders down to his knees. The dry salt causes a circulation pick-up and sends streams of vitality shooting through his tired body. He thrills to this dry salt rub and feels his tensions melting with the dissolved salt in the water. Then he rinses with *cool* water and he greets the day with youthful energy.

GRECIAN HERBAL BATH   Here is an herbal-vinegar bath that was said to have made Helen of Troy the legendary beauty with the face that launched a thousand ships. Take two drams each of these herbs: rosemary, lavender, rue and also camphor; soak in one pint of white wine vinegar for a few hours. Strain off the herbs. Now pour the liquid into the comfortably warm bath water and soak your way to Grecian beauty.

HERB RUBDOWN   The sluggish nerves of the skin are often in need of a brisk alerting. Here is an historical herbal compound that can help pep up the lazy skin cells and awaken the nerve responses.

Mix these ingredients together: 1 cup finely ground oatmeal; 3 ounces almond meal; 1 cake castile soap, finely shaved; 1/4 lb. powdered orris root (this has a tingly violet fragrance). Put in cheese cloth bags. Following a tub bath, rub yourself with this Herbal Bag instead of a wash cloth. You'll glow all over!

BUBBLY OXYGEN BATH   This water healing secret of the past has an unsual "aeration" benefit. It helps restore oxygen depletion to the system, thus "feeding" the bloodstream with much needed air. Many who complain of chronic exhaustion, tiredness, short-windedness and habitual mouth-breathing because of respiratory difficulties, should consider this time-tested folk healer. Here's how to self-oxygenate with a Bubbly Oxygen Bath:

Sprinkle 20 tablespoons of sodium perborate on the surface of a tub of warm water. Add 2 tablespoons of manganese borate and

4 tablespoons of ordinary baking soda. In a few seconds, oxygen begins to be given off and continues for twenty minutes. It is said to be as refreshingly good as a bubbly champagne bath—and lots cheaper, too! Ingredients are available at most pharmacies.

HOT AND COLD WATER "SOAKS" FOR HEALTH STIMULATION

The ancients and even the moderns called it *hydrotherapy* or healing with water. Our ancestors used cold water as a reviving procedure. It still is the first thing used to revive a person in a faint. Cold has a naturally stimulating process. From this humble beginning, hydrotherapy has developed into a time-tested and natural healer.

Water Stimulates Nerve Health

A great many nerves end on the body surface; among them nerve endings for heat and cold. There are separate receptors for heat and cold, hence the importance of *contrast* soaks. Folk healing called for alternate soaks to help revive sluggish or weak nerves.

CONTRAST "SOAKS" FOR HAND WARMING   Folks who kept wringing cold hands would follow this natural healer. Soak both hands in comfortably hot water for several moments. Then remove and plunge into cold water for several moments. Continue the Contrast "Soaks" for a dozen times. Always begin and end with the warm soak. The hands (and feet, too, may be warmed with the Contrast "Soaks") slowly take on a soothing warmth.

Benefits of Hot Water

The secret benefits of hot water lie in the relaxation of smooth-muscle cells. Blood flow is slowed because the amount of circulating blood is not varied from minute to minute. Slowing of the blood causes the amount of blood in the hands to become larger. This blood increase creates a feeling of comforting warmth. Reportedly, discomforting pain at the soaked site is lessened and soothing relaxation is provided.

How Cold Soaks Revitalize Circulation

Many of the proponents of water healing emphasized cold soaks to those who could comfortably take them. The benefits reported include the "goose flesh" of the skin. So-called "goose flesh" is caused by constriction of the small blood vessels and contraction of the muscular and elastic tissues in and under the skin. Just a brief Cold Soak causes the constricted blood vessels to immediately dilate again; more blood flows through and the skin becomes pink and warm. Generally, a sensation of revitalized circulation and general stimulation is enjoyed.

FOMENTATIONS: ANCIENT WATER APPLICATION

A fomentation is a local application of hot and cold, applied alternately to promote relaxation of spasms, to pep up a lazy circulation, to reduce symptomatic reactions of swelling and to provide a feeling of general well-being. It was popular in the days of the ancient health-conscious Greeks who would nurse aching joints and throbbing pains with fomentations.

How to Make a Fomentation

Take one-half of a single bed cotton blanket and fold twelve inches wide. Take one-half of a single woolen blanket. Have a large pan with boiling water. Dip the cotton blanket in it up to three or four inches of the ends; the water must be boiling hot.

Wring the folded blanket out of the water; spread a flannel blanket out on a table. Put the steaming cotton blanket on it, folding twice on one side and once on the other.

Now apply to the ailing region or to the portion that needs to benefit from this ancient folk healer. Leave on until it is cool. Then remove. Repeat for a half dozen applications.

Professionals suggest that this series of fomentations be applied for a period of from fifteen minutes to one hour. Many clinicians have reported that fomentations help in conditions of local pains and congestion and soothe symptoms of neuralgia and problems of aching joints.

Where to Apply Fomentations

Professionals suggest applications to be made on the *surrounding* portion of the body that needs help. If there is a difficult-to-reach portion, ask a family member to help.

HOW WATER SOOTHES BACK-SHOULDER DISTRESS

For muscular stiffness of the low back, here are two reported pain-easers by means of Nature's gift—water:

HOT SHALLOW TUB   Fill a tub with four inches of hot but not scalding (about 112°F) water. Lie on your back in the warm water. Keep your feet flat against the wall above the foot end of the tub or rest your heels on the tub's rim. Slowly, inch down toward the foot of the tub so your legs are bent more and more sharply. Slowly, you will feel a gentle relaxation of your back muscles. Simultaneously, stretch from the hip-rolling action of this leg position. About ten minutes should help give healing hot water an opportunity to soothe your stiff back.

HOT SHOWER WITH SPINE-ROLLING   Stand in the tub, your back toward the water. Keep legs slightly apart and knees slightly bent. Place both hands on your knees. Support the upper part of your body with your arms. Adjust a hot shower spray upon your back. Arch your lower segment. Raise first one hip, then the other in slow precision, working your back muscles gently and smoothly while shower heat helps loosen and soothe congestion. Permit this natural water healer about fifteen minutes to do its reportedly relaxing benefit.

We have come a long way since the days of Poppaea Sabina, the wife of Nero. She would bathe daily in milk; she had a drove of 500 female mules shod with gold, to furnish milk for this purpose. Today, baths are more private and prosaic, and certainly most healing. Water is more than Nature's cleansing treasure. It is Nature's own healer!

MAIN BENEFITS IN SUMMARY

1. Steam helps wash and scrub the arteries, restoring lubrication and elasticity to cholesterol-covered lifelines of the body.
2. A Hot Tub–Cold Shower Energizer helps put life into a tired mind and body.
3. Simple Moist Abdominal Wraparound applied nightly helps establish digestive youth.
4. Skin is healthfully improved with water. Tensions reportedly can be rubbed away with ordinary salt.

5. Take a tip from the beautiful Greeks and enjoy a Grecian Herbal Bath as well as a Herb Rubdown. Do it to yourself.
6. Improve body's oxygen with a folk healing Bubbly Oxygen Bath.
7. Contrast soaks help soothe nerves, warm hands, revitalize circulation.
8. Fomentations are ancient water healing applications to soothe swelling and aching joints.
9. Ease low back congestion with a Hot Shallow Tub and a Hot Shower With Spine-Rolling folk healing secret.

9

"Exer-Breathing"—
Natural Key to Internal Cleansing

Each morning, Martin L. gives himself an "air wash." Through many published reports by leading physical therapists and physicians, Martin L. has learned that proper self-ventilation and self-cleansing helps "scrub" out the accumulated wastes, toxemia and infectious debris that is known to cling to the respiratory organs. Thanks to healthful living and the following four early-morning Exer-Breathing exercises, he has strengthened his breathing apparatus and is able to resist the ravages of allergic offenders. Martin L. also conquered chronic sniffles and a feeling of tiredness by taking a tip from the ancient yogis, who were thousands of years ahead of their time by advocating Exer-Breathing.

Following are the four Exer-Breathing exercises that Martin L. performs each morning as a means of air washing his insides. (Internal cleanliness is as important as, if not more than, external cleanliness.)

1. In the open air, or with windows open, stand with hands on the lower ribs.

2. Breathe in slowly through the nostrils, and be sure the *lower* ribs are being pushed out. Many people breathe without using the lower rib muscles to their fullest capacity. It will take practice to accomplish it.

3. At the end of breathing *in* (inspiration), after taking in all the air it seems possible, take in *another breath*. Then take one

more. As you take in the last whiff, hook your fingers under your ribs and give them a tug outward.

4. Now with mouth open, let all the air out, and at the end of expiration push the lower ribs *in*. Grunt to get the last bit of air out. Do the above Exer-Breathing in the morning, to give yourself an air wash just as you give yourself an outside washing. It helps sweep away the cobwebs of sluggishness and invigorates the system for the tasks of the day ahead.

(*For variety:* breathe in rapidly and expel the air slowly, or breathe in very slowly and exhale rapidly. You may also raise the arms slowly up over the head while breathing in. This helps expand the rib cage.)

Reported benefits of Exer-Breathing include better sleeping, better appetite, improved circulation and a pepped up thinking capacity. In short, Exer-Breathing helps you start on a new way of better living.

HOW EXER-BREATHING CAN HELP INTERNAL FITNESS

Oxygen is the life's blood of all body cells. You have some 750 million air sacs or cells, through which precious oxygen passes to get into the bloodstream. At any given second, one quarter of the blood contained in the human body passes over the surface area of the lungs to give up the carbon dioxide gas that it is carrying. The blood then takes on oxygen from the air ingested for the return circuit back to the cells.

Oxygen Improves Thinking Power

By means of Exer-Breathing, this ancient yogi-inspired self-ventilation process is able to nourish the brain. The cells which are most sensitive to oxygen shortage are the brain cells. Most people who have sluggish thinking would do well to look to the ancients who would use natural air to help send a fresh and invigorating flow of oxygen into the bloodstream to electrify the entire system. Exer-Breathing sends valuable oxygen to the higher centers of the brain to influence reasoning, will power and judgment.

A DESK-BOUND EXECUTIVE BREATHES WAY TO FITNESS

Louis J. felt "old" at 51. It began when he experienced what a neighbor called "middle-age breathlessness." He would grow tired after a short walk around the block. In addition to so-called "loss of wind," Louis felt tense and upset. He had a feeling of fullness in his digestive system. He was embarrassed by a slight bulge at the middle. What really won him over to Exer-Breathing was his night gasping. When he would lie flat on the bed at night, he would frequently experience such shortness of breath, he had to get up and go to the window for more air. Physically, he appeared to be healthy. But Louis wanted to do something about his condition.

Diaphragm Is Key to Internal Cleanliness

Louis learned that the ancients as well as practitioners of yogi and modern-day jogging or aerobics, were aware of the influence of the diaphragm on overall health. This is the "bottom of the bellows" which divides the lungs from the abdominal cavity. This muscular sheet works by moving from a high, arched position up inside the chest to a flat disc at its bottom. With advancing years, some of the elasticity of the lungs (as with the skin) begins to weaken. This is Nature's signal that internal cleanliness is at stake.

Louis J. was able to help strengthen the diaphragm even though he rarely left his desk. He performed this reported Exer-Breathing motion as often as possible throughout the day:

SELF-CLEANSING DIAPHRAGM EXER-BREATHING   Sit erect in a straight chair. Place both hands flat on the lower chest and upper abdomen, with about one hand's breadth dividing them. Take a normal breath. Let it out. When the end of the normal exhalation is felt, press with both hands to expel as much more air as possible. About every third breath, press very vigorously and sharply, in the equivalent of a false cough.

(*Benefit:* the secret reported benefit of this modern adaptation of an ancient Eastern-Oriental Exer-Breathing motion is to milk mucus out of the pockets in your respiratory system and to help "squeeze" out the wastes that cling to the lungs. This helps cleanse and "scrub" the filters of your lungs, benefiting your body with a fresh supply of nourishing oxygen.)

FOR SELF-CLEANSING PLUS   Keep your hands as flat as if they were pressing on a table top—if you let your fingers dig in even a little bit, they may cause sore muscles. Continue for about a dozen breaths. Repeat three times daily. Reported benefits include easing of the ravages of asthma, bronchitis, emphysema and other chest disorders. Here we see how accumulated sludge may be the forerunner of respiratory conditions. Air-washing is simple, free and puts life into your lungs!

Louis J. managed to obtain relief from his disorders; then he gave up the Exer-Breathing and his over-confidence led to a serious bout with allergic super-sensitivity. Much later, in combination with proper foods, rest and relaxation, Exer-Breathing helped put him in Nature's balanced health. Louis J. learned from the ancients and from folk healing emphasis upon breathing that it must be performed regularly for overall benefit.

TWO SIMPLE EXER-BREATHING STEPS TO YOUTHFUL VITALITY

Joanne R. took a trip to India. Here she found endless people in substandard living conditions. But Joanne R. saw that there were many octogenarians who performed the work of young people. Joanne was in her late 50's and already resigned to doing easier work with less responsibility. She always felt her youth was slipping. Yet, she saw these oldsters carrying heavy bundles, working in the fields from dawn to dusk, with no noticeable signs of "civilized exhaustion." What was their secret?

Joanne Learns About "Youth Breathing"

She talked to university students and was told that many of the natives of India and the entire region surrounding, were followers of the ancient practice of *pranayama*. Rich or poor, they used these breathing exercises as a means of relieving internal obstructions. This was one reason for their apparent good physical health.

"Youth Breathing" is an apt identification for such historic practices that are most prominent today. Currently, we see the emergence of special yogi schools in our civilized world. Many have reported a feeling of youth restoration by special "Youth Breathing" and overall natural-cleansing living.

Joanne followed these Youth Breathing exercises when she came home:

1. Close one nostril with the fingers; breathe in, using sniffs, through the other nostril. Now, close the second nostril, exhale, and then breathe in, using sniffs, through the other nostril. Alternate up to ten times. This exercise reportedly clears the sinus region and helps cleanse this filtering area.

2. While walking, or in any position, force air out in short breaths through pursed lips in a shush or whistle to a tune of some kind. Inhale in short sniffs forcibly snuffing in through your nose. This Youth Breathing exercise is a basis of yoga and reportedly helps to exhale the toxic sludge from the body.

3. Lie down or sit back in a comfortable chair that supports your back. Relax your chest and abdomen completely. Now suck in your abdomen sharply, forcing air out through your nose or mouth. Relax your abdomen, reinflating your lungs. Devote one second to each phase, so that continuous breathing in this way involves about 30 breaths a minute—half again the usual relaxed breathing rate. Continue for three minutes. Many laboring Indian yoga devotees will use this exercise as a means of helping to oxygenate and ventilate the tired respiratory system.

Joanne Feels and Looks Younger Through Youth Breathing

By following several of the breathing programs as well as general dietary improvements which called for elimination of artificial foods, desserts, rich gravies, excessively sweet and spiced items, Joanne R. experienced a rejuvenation that made her feel and look younger. She follows Youth Breathing programs as a "health tonic" to keep herself in a self-cleansed condition. Her trip to India had, literally, given her a new lease on life!

JOGGING HELPS INTERNAL METABOLISM

As a simple exercise, jogging reportedly has the most phenomenal benefits. Jogging, simply put, is running at your own pace. It helps cause an invigoration of the respiratory system and thereby helps internal metabolism. It reportedly helps increase the blood flow to the heart, firm and tone up the muscles, invigorate circulation, and strengthen the action of the other vital body processes.

Join Local Physical Fitness Groups

While you may like to jog alone, there is always comfort and security in crowds. Jogging in groups is interesting and offers companionship. Inquire at your local Health Department for information about such groups.

Jog Your Way to Natural Oxygenation

Overall, balanced movement helps send streams of fresh oxygen throughout the system. To jog, you start at a speedy walk, increase your pace to a comfortable running. When you begin to feel a little tired or breathless, you slow down to a walk. You keep moving while you're resting. When you've had a chance to get your breath back, you start the speedy walk and then the gradually increasing running gait.

EASY STEPS TO JOGGING   To enable the benefits of jogging to perform their health building, here are reported suggestions:

Posture. While walking or running, stand up straight. Keep your head up. Keep your back as straight as is natural and comfortable.

Arm Movements. Your elbows should be kept slightly bent and away from your body. Let them move rhythmically forward and back.

Leg Movements. Move your legs from your hips with an easy and unforced action. Lift from your knees while you keep your ankles relaxed. Do not reach out for a long stride. Rather, let each step take you a comfortably normal distance.

Breathing. Inhale as much air as possible through your nose and your mouth. You need to wash your system with fresh oxygen. This is one of the greatest reported benefits of jogging.

Footstrike. Land on your heel and roll forward onto your toe before that leg takes off again. This heel-to-toe method is least tiring over long distances and minimizes strain. If this type of footstriking is uncomfortable, then you may adopt your own method.

You may jog on any flat surface: a regulation cinder track, a neighborhood sidewalk, park or field, even in an office. When outdoors, you can find country roads, beaches, vacant lots or any suitable surface. The most ideal area is a spacious grassy one because the softness of the ground is easier on the ankle and knee joints.

OXYGEN: STAFF OF LIFE

The ancients who emphasized breathing were unaware of the technical benefits but were very much aware of its overall benefits. Oxygen, the elixir of life, is long known to be one of the best blood purifiers and one of the most effective nerve tonics. This staff of life is amply provided by Nature for all. By exhaling the poisonous waste matters, the circulatory system becomes washed, the respiratory system enjoys a fresh cleansing, digestion becomes subsequently improved, the skin develops a healthy glow and the mental outlook is sparked with youthful vitality. Take a tip from the health secrets of the Orient and East—"Exer-Breathe" for internal cleanliness.

SUMMARY

1. Morning Exer-Breathing helps replenish lost oxygen and creates internal washing.
2. Simple Eastern-Oriental Exer-Breathing motions help milk mucus out of the pockets in the respiratory system.
3. Desk-bound folks benefit from easy Self-Cleansing without leaving their work.
4. *Pranayama*—India-created Exer-Breathing is a form of Youth Breathing.
5. Jogging is the easy way to replenish the system with oxygen: staff of life.

10

How Nature Can Bestow
a Healthful Sleep

A good night's sleep becomes more and more healthful to you as you get older. Youthful sleep helps rest the body's systems, replenish the mind, and create natural healing processes to invigorate the senses. Sleep may be considered Nature's healing tonic.

Look to Nature for Natural Herbal Sleeping Potions

In the vast array of folklore healing medicines from the meadows, there are herbs which were used by pioneers, the hardy Indians, and early settlers. (They, too, had occasional sleeping problems and would look to Nature for help.)

Sleep-Ease Herbs

The following herbs are reportedly effective in helping create a drowsy and sleepy feeling: lady's slipper, valerian, scullcap and hops. Use one teaspoonful of any *one* of these herbs; steep in a cup of boiling water twenty minutes and drink piping hot. Folklore herbalists sang the praises of these herbs which they said would soothe the nerves and create a relaxing tonic to the entire system. (Sleeping pills, aspirin, bromides, etc., work by deadening the nerves; they also leave harsh chemicalized caustic reactions to the sensitive body tissues.)

HERBAL SLEEP-TIGHT TONIC   Through word of mouth, Indians kept alive the secret of a special all-natural sleeping tonic. Early western explorers were able to learn the secret formula which consists of herbs gathered from the fields. Today, most herbalists can supply the valuable healing grasses. The Indians would mix equal parts of these herbs: scullcap, nerve root, hops, black cohosh. They would stir them together and then steep one teaspoonful in a cup of boiling water just fifteen minutes. Then they would sip slowly. This Herbal Sleep-Tight Tonic reportedly relaxed the nerves and enabled the tired person to enjoy a healthful and natural sleep.

HOW TO RELAX YOUR WAY TO RESTFUL SLEEP

Marcia D. is a bundle of nerves. She is so tensed up, she snaps at friends and family, loses her temper with the delivery men, and is a fright to live with! Overwrought, Marcia cannot get a good night's sleep. She tosses and turns until early dawn and even then she cannot get in enough sleep. Marcia might have headed for an inevitable nervous breakdown or emotional collapse had not a relative insisted she try self-relaxation.

This relative had once been troubled by insomnia and sought help from natural healers. They taught her the art of "letting go" in a series of amazingly simple twist-and-ease motions.

Marcia scoffed, but her nerves were so "fit to be tied" that she eventually submitted to the natural ways of relaxing tight muscles and inducing sleep. Here is what Marcia did, based upon suggestions by natural healers:

TWIST 'N' EASE RELAXING MOTIONS   These relaxing and sleep-inducing motions are best done while lying on the back.

1. Clench both fists. Notice the pull or tenseness on your wrist, around your elbow, and even up in the shoulder. This is extreme muscular tension.

2. Open your fists. Immediately the muscles of hand, forearm, arm and shoulder release their contraction—and in so doing, tension is gone.

3. Perform the above motion three times; clench and relax three times.

4. Next, bend the toes and feet downward, and push or stretch downward with the heels. Notice the pull or tenseness in your ankles, feet, hips and thighs, but especially in the calves of the legs. This is muscular tension.

5. Now let go and the muscular tension is "milked" away.

6. Do the foot exercise three times. Repeat Nos. 4 and 5 three times.

7. This last relaxing motion is for the muscles of the neck, throat and face. First, close the eyes. Shut them as tightly as you can. At the same time press the lips together and bite hard with the jaws. This contracts the muscles of your eyes, forehead, mouth, jaw and neck. You can easily feel the tension about the head—and even hear it ringing in your ears.

8. Now let go with your jaw and face. If your head falls to one side, let it. You are learning to release tension, learning to relax your way to sleep.

9. Perform the face and jaw motions three times (Nos. 7 and 8). You may need to practice many times on this last exercise before you feel the benefits because, of all the body muscles, those in the face are often among the most difficult to learn how to relax. Check yourself sometime when you are unable to sleep, and you will often find your eyebrows knit together, your forehead wrinkled up and the muscles around the eyes and jaws tense.

Gradual Relief Soothes Marcia

It took a few days of practice of the above routine until Marcia became more relaxed, soothed. She did admit to a pleasurable sense of "all-goneness" after doing the exercise and this helped bring her blessed sleep. Now Marcia became a rational person to live with. She liked others and they liked her. She soon liked herself!

HOW WATER HELPS PROMOTE SLEEP

By immersing one's self in a warm tub, there is a general feeling of absolute relaxation. The heat helps numb the delicate nerve endings and soothe frazzled raw edges. This time-honored sleep-inducement is as helpful today as it always was. Benefits are greater if you will *not* rub yourself vigorously with a towel after the bath; that stimulates the nerve ends and may cause insomnia. Dry yourself by patting the towel against your body. This is soothing, like the mother's gentle pat which calms her baby into a lulling sleep.

How Moist Heat Relaxes "Insomnia Spots"

Poor Jennifer maintained that it was bad enough to feel tense and "knotty," but what really kept her awake most of the night was what she called "insomnia spots." These were extremely "tight" regions of her body, in localized areas such as the neck, shoulders, small of the back, and the spine. These often set up a strange chain reaction that kept her awake all night.

Jennifer followed Grandma's program of using *moist heat* to help ease and soothe those "insomnia spots." This helped Jennifer, but she was an habitual worrier and, if it wasn't one thing it was another that kept her tossing and turning. Eventually, she took barbiturates and a near-fatality spurred her back to Grandma's *moist heat* applications for those "insomnia spots" and also spurred Jennifer to soothe her worried nature. Here's how moist heat relaxes "insomnia spots":

Soak a large bath towel in hot water. Wring it out and place it on the tense, congested area. To retain the heat longer, cover the towel with another dry towel, plus a small blanket over all this to retain the heat.

A 15-minute moist heat application is reportedly wonderfully relaxing and helps ease the tight, tense muscles of the neck and shoulders and those along the spine. Once these muscles "let go" through the action of moist heat applications, sleep is welcome in its arrival.

HOT FOOT BATH IS NATURE'S SLEEP TREATMENT   Ever since we can remember, a natural sleep-relaxant was a hot foot bath. It's as effective as ever. Soak the feet in hot water for 15 minutes. The benefit here is that the heat serves to improve circulation by sending blood tingling through the blood vessels. This relieves tension, restores a normal circulation and induces a feeling of relaxation.

Finish the foot bath by pouring cool water over the feet. Dry thoroughly, particularly between the toes. Massage the feet and ankles and calves upward toward the heart with rubbing alcohol. Then, enjoy a good night's sleep.

HOW RELAXED EYES INDUCE RELAXED SLEEP

Brain workers are often insomniacs because their eyes are subjected to such strain that even when their lids are closed in sleep, the eyes tend to stare straight ahead. This leads to a fatigued feeling when awakening.

WATER APPLICATIONS RELIEVE EYE FATIGUE   To relax the eyes and let them sleep, a simple time-honored folk healer calls for the application of comfortably hot water to soothe the eye muscles, followed by an application of cold water to refresh them.

Soak a washcloth in comfortably hot water and apply to the eyes for two minutes. Then take another washcloth, soak in comfortably cold water and apply to the eyes. This contrast water application was used by insomnia-folks in the days before barbiturates and sleeping pills. Water applications are all-natural! Pills, on the other hand, interfere with your ability to relax and sleep spontaneously. They are a crutch; they are not remedial because they do not remove the cause of insomnia. Small wonder that folk healers looked to Nature for giving them a soothing night's sleep.

HOW PERSIANS INDUCED PLEASING SLEEP

Royalists of the ancient Persian courts had their problems; in the midst of luxuries, they were constantly beset with political tensions, intrigues and the rigors of revolution. Folklore tells us that the Persian rulers almost always enjoyed a good night's sleep because they followed a special program. Its origin is lost in history but its effect is apparently as welcome as always.

Sleeping on the Right Side

The Persian would sleep on the *right* side. Today, modern practitioners feel this is the best sleeping side because the work of the heart, lungs and the stomach is unimpeded since they are on the top of other inner organs in this position. It is advisable to change your sleeping position a few times during the night.

Omit Pillows for Healthful Sleep

The Persian who had insomnia would eliminate any pillow. The reason? Today we have learned that sleeping on high pillows strains the neck and causes curvature of the spine. They also tend to lessen flow of blood to the head.

BABYLONIAN BREATHING-TO-SLEEP SECRET   The sages and wise men of Babylon were hired by Persian rulers to teach them the sacred secrets of healthful sleep. They believed that sleep could be induced by invoking a goddess. The wise men taught the chosen few rulers a rather simple but amazingly effective way to Breathe-Sleep. Here's how:

Breathe *in* through the mouth. Breathe *out* through the nose. Continue doing so as the feeling of well-being comes over the senses and a healthful sleep is induced.

How Breathing-to-Sleep Benefits Health

The Babylonian natural healers lacked our modern scientific laboratories and thus were unable to create habit-forming drugs and symptom-causing chemical medicines. They looked to Nature for healing and while they could not use scientific jargon to explain how Breathing-to-Sleep benefits, they accepted it. This technique was effective and all-natural.

Today, we know that this works because breathing activates the thermostatic control mechanism that is comprised of nerve centers, or ganglia of the sympathetic and parasympathetic nervous systems as well as a vast plexus of nerve fibers. These connect the centers with the blood vessels and nerve supply of every part of the body.

The Breathing-to-Sleep Program activates this function and sends a fresh wave of soothing oxygen to all nerve fibers, helping to nourish and relax them. Sleep is close behind after nerve relaxation.

YAWN YOUR WAY TO SLEEP

The mouth is often the most tense part of the face. Drop your jaws down, continue to drop them until you go into a yawn. Yawning is one of the most natural and beneficial inducements toward sleep. Open your mouth wide, draw in air to capacity, pushing down on your diaphragm and stretching apart all the bones and muscles of your head and neck. Continue doing so until you feel a gradual relaxation. Just let go—and go to sleep!

SUMMARY

1. Folk healers relied upon herbs in a tasty tea to help create natural sleep. Herbs are Nature's oldest natural sleeping tonics.

2. Twist 'N' Ease Relaxing Motions help take the kinks and knots out of the body and pave the way for restful sleep.
3. Moist heat applications relax "insomnia spots" and erase tensions.
4. Relaxed eyes promote general contentment and a sleep environment. Water applications have soothed tired eyes since time immemorial.
5. Take a tip from the Persians on right side sleeping; omit pillows for spinal health.
6. Babylonian Breathing-to-Sleep Secret is now available for modern utilization.

II

How the American Indians Used Natural Remedies for Strong Eyesight

Long before the appearance of the covered wagon, the golden West was a treasure of healing herbs and Nature-grown grasses and ferns. The Indians who roamed the plains were vigorous, healthy, and totally dependent upon Nature for its healing sources. The Indians knew nothing of civilized laboratories and patent medicines; they relied exclusively upon the secrets of Nature for healing and soothing. They were rewarded by Nature with magnificent bodies, longevity (most Indians lived well up to the age of 100), and remarkable freedom from so-called diseases of civilization.

The Indians were also rewarded by Nature with strong and healthy eyesight. Early missionary doctors who ventured into savage Indian camps and were able to make friends with these devotees of Nature, reported that their eyes were unusually strong, healthy and free from the problems of squint, near and far-sightedness, blurring, ache, dim vision and other current disorders.

Indians Used Herbs for Visual Strengthening

The American Indian put full faith on the floral medicines of forest and field to alleviate his ills and to strengthen his sight. He knew that his very life depended upon strong eyesight. When the early colonists came to the New World, they brought with them some knowledge of herbs and natural sight-strengtheners, only to learn that the Indians had been using them for many generations.

The Red Man's close affinity with Nature was rewarded with strong eyesight and overall vigorous health to combat the elements and the ravages of severe climate, rough terrain, constant outdoor living, and privation and struggle that claimed the lives of the early colonists. The Indian was able to survive because he relied almost entirely upon the plant kingdom for his medicinal needs. He was able to possess powerful sight and hearing by means of herbal strengthening.

THE SIGHT-IMPROVING HERB
OF THE SIOUX INDIANS

The Sioux Indians lived in the midwest, roaming over plains of rich herbs and medicinal plants. They reportedly would gather a herb aptly called *golden seal*. This was a small perennial plant, that grew a gold-colored flower. It flourished in the moist, rich woodlands. Because it bears a seal-like scar on the yellow-gold root, herbalists and botanists called it golden seal. The Sioux Indians reportedly would gather this herb, boil it in water and then use it as an eye wash. Early colonists reported the Sioux would use the golden seal eye wash before a battle. Apparently, they placed much value in its sight-strengthening properties. Today, modern herbalists offer this Indian-based eye-strengthener with these suggestions:

Take one teaspoon golden seal, one level teaspoon boric acid, dissolve in a pint of boiling water. Shake well. Let settle. Pour off the liquid, let it cool, and use in eye cups to refresh and cleanse the eyes.

THE HERB THAT STRENGTHENED
THE EYES OF THE CHEYENNE

The Cheyenne Indians were known for their excellent health and stamina. They also fought, though unsuccessfully, the invading colonists when other Indians succumbed and surrendered. The Cheyenne lived in the much-cherished land along the Santa Fe and Platte River trails that were used by the settlers on their way to California and Oregon. Here, the plant kingdom flourished.

Here, the Cheyenne used *fennel seed and leaves* for remarkable sight-strengthening properties.

Benefits of Fennel

As a healing herb, fennel is beneficial for soothing problems of insect bites and scratches, skin irritations, visual disturbances. The Cheyenne were ahead of the colonists in using fennel for strong sight and overall health.

FENNEL EYE WASH   Herbalists suggest a daily eyewash that is made by soaking one teaspoon of fennel seed and/or leaves in a cup of boiled water. Strain. Then use as an eyewash with an eye cup. The soothing qualities offer relaxation to tired eyes. Tension is frequently the cause of eye strain and eye decline so the herbal way to sight improvement is through relaxation. The Cheyenne would gather fennel from the woods and always keep a fresh supply available for soothing their precious eyesight.

THE EYE-HEALING SECRET
OF THE NEZ PERCÉS

The Nez Percés welcomed and aided the Lewis and Clark expedition which crossed their northwestern lands in 1805. Journals left by these explorers tell of their remarkable eye health, as well as robust physical condition. The Nez Percés were long known for exceptionally strong eyesight and, when colonists inquired, they were told that the herbs of Nature gave them health.

Chronicles and journals of that era tell of learning the secret herbs used by the Nez Percés and how these medicines from the plant kingdom served to nourish and strengthen the eyesight.

HERBS FOR "INDIAN-STRONG" EYES   These Nature-loving Indians would use the following eye wash: Steep one teaspoon of red raspberry leaves, one teaspoon witch hazel leaves in a cup of boiling water. Strain through a cloth. Saturate a soft cloth with this herbal tea and apply as a wet pack to the eyes. Bathe the eyes often with this herbal wash, as did the Nez Percés who never wore glasses!

THE HERB THAT SOOTHES EYE INFLAMMATION

In a pioneer paper, *The Prescott Miner,* published in the 1860's, reference is made to a simple herb poultice used by the

Apache Indians for healing of wounds, lacerations, injuries and, particularly, eye inflammation. It was written that the Apache medicine man would roam the trails, canyons and crevices of the Southwest, to gather what we today call *slippery elm.*

This herb has a soothing and "slippery" action that helps draw out the infectious wastes and restore a sense of health and visual comfort. The Apaches would take slippery elm bark, soak in boiled water, then wrap in a bit of cloth, apply as a poultice to tired, inflamed, itchy, grainy or otherwise ailing eyes. They would let remain for a half hour or longer. They would repeat this slippery elm poultice at frequent intervals until the visual inflammation and tiredness was eased. Reportedly, the Apaches had superior vision and Nature rewarded them with its bountiful treasures of healing from the plant kingdom.

Today, slippery elm is available at most herbalists and there is no need to go gather it in the mountains of the once-flourishing Indian country.

INDIAN-INSPIRED EYE HEALERS

Based upon folklore healing reports among the sight-strong Indians, other natural methods include these:

HOW TEA REFRESHES TIRED EYES   Our great-grandmothers learned this secret from the Indians. Soak gauze pads in weak herbal tea. Lie down for at least thirty minutes with the gauze pads on the eyes. This rests and brightens the eyes.

EYE TENSION RELAXATION   Steep green tea in rose water. Soak absorbent cotton pads and then apply to the eyes while lying down for thirty minutes.

THE PIONEER EYE WASH   Soak cotton pads in witch hazel and apply to the eyes while lying down. The pioneers would become soothed and refreshed with this natural eye wash.

CHEROKEE EYE WASH HEALER   Colonists and journal-keepers told of a powder used by the Cherokees for soothing inflamed, infected and diseased eyes. Later, it was found that the powder was a crude form of our more modern boric acid. The healing eye wash is made by pouring a little boric acid into boiling water. When comfortably cool, use with an eye cup. The Cherokees took their crude form of boric acid powder wherever they went. Nature rewarded them with healthy eyes.

WET TEA BAGS REJUVENATE EYES   Joan C., a film star who is constantly subjected to the glaring lights of the camera and the heat of the artificial sunlamps while making pictures, tells of her discovery for eye health—she takes two wet tea bags (herbal tea bags are recommended) and puts them on the eyes while she rests for thirty minutes. Joan C. keeps her eyes healthy, strong and refreshed with this simple herbal folk healer.

HOT CLOTHS HEAL EYE DISTRESS   A physician who believes in looking to Nature for sight care, suggests a folk healing program that uses hot cloths:

Fold an ordinary washcloth to four layers' thickness. Dip in water which is as hot as is comfortable (112°F) and wring partially dry. Apply to eye, and cover with a dry towel to help hold the heat. Change as often as necessary to keep the cloth hot for twenty minutes.

WATER: NATURAL EYE WASH

Why Water Is Healthful to Eyes

A great part of the eye and its fluids and tissues are water. Water as an eye wash, especially in the hot and/or cold applications, has a "pumping" action on the circulation; first the water expands tissues and fluid contents especially, and secondly the blood lymph plus interstitial fluids (fluid lying between the cells). This helps improve congestion. The Indians and others who discovered the healing power of water would greatly benefit by simple water washing.

WATER APPLICATIONS EASE VISUAL CONGESTION   Nightly, Michael M. would soak cloths in comfortably hot water. He would apply the comfortably warm cloths to his eyes. Then, after thirty minutes, he would soak cloths in comfortably cold water and take a half hour eye soak. This helped soothe Michael's nervous eye tremors and also restored some of his dimming vision.

Underwater Blinking Improves Visual Strength

The eyes can be winked and blinked under water in a wide open basin, or two basins, with different temperatures. The benefit here is that underwater blinking removes mucous from the eyes, washes away powdered dirt from the lids and eyelashes; also, washing off the cornea makes the eyes feel fresh. One can sometimes feel a freshening of sight and a possible fraction of improved sight may result a short time after cleansing action.

Alternate Water Baths for Visual Cleansing

Contrast or alternate cold and warm water washings have always been known to the early colonists and the so-called primitive Indians. Today, we know that, according to physics, heat causes expansion and cold causes contraction. This alternate water washing has a self-cleansing action on visual congestion. This congestion may be traced to abuse of overworked blood vessels, or a too-viscid bloodstream content caused by accumulation of too many waste substances, as well as a slow, stagnant circulation. Alternate water baths may be applied by the conventional eye cup, your palms, or just use wash cloths. Alternate cold and warm Water Baths help cleanse out the infectious wastes and corrosive acids that may accumulate in visual arteries and vessels and impede healthful sight. The Indians had the right idea. They sought out Nature for visual health and never needed eyeglasses!

HOW EXERCISE CORRECTS VISUAL DISCOMFORTS

Use, but *do not abuse,* your eyes! Since the eye is a muscle, it needs proper exercise. Here are nine reported visual correction exercises that are beneficial for the eyes:

1. Sit in a chair completely relaxed. Move your eyes slowly in a wide circle, first several times in one direction, then slowly in the opposite one.

2. Move your eyes as far to the left and then as far to the right as possible.

3. Do the same up and down, also far to the right top corner and to the bottom left corner; next to the left top corner and the bottom right one.

4. Rub the palms of your hands on one another to produce electricity and then cover your eyes with them. Many folk healers maintain this causes a self-generating electrolyte reaction that supercharges the eyes with natural vitality.

5. Gently rub your eyes with your knuckles, in a manner similar to that you may have observed a cat doing this relaxing routine.

6. Here is an exercise claimed to be quite beneficial—look far away. Then suddenly, look very near you as at the point of your nose and then back again. Repeat this routine several times whenever you feel your eyes to be tense or overly rigid.

7. Blink your eyelids frequently during the day, at work, while reading or walking. This relaxes the eyes, washes and lubricates them with the tear fluid secreted by the tear glands.

8. Alternate hot and cold wet towel applications to improve the circulation of the blood to the eyes.

9. Look frequently at pleasant, natural things such as trees, meadows, foilage, grass, all of Nature. It did well for the Indians!

RELAX YOUR WAY TO SIGHT HEALTH

Never stare at objects, because that is a strain for the eyes. Always keep your eyes moving and blink your eyelids wherever you are. This helps induce relaxation, the key to better sight.

FOREHEAD COMPRESSION FOR SIGHT SOOTHING   Many who have used deep compression therapy or reflexology have advocated this simple drugless method of relieving pressure that may cause tired eyes:

While lying in bed, lace your fingers together. Place your palms on your forehead. Slightly gather the skin of your forehead. Let the weight of the hands be toward your eyes, and not toward the back of your head. Your hands should be so braced by the lacing of your fingers that they do not separate. Let your elbows fall back on the bed. Thus, your forehead receives the full weight of your hands. Maintain this forehead compression for fifteen minutes or until sight tension is felt melting.

Look to Nature for Sight Health

The Indians and other primitives who sought sight health would look to Nature in the form of herbs, special water washes and self-massages. Remember that your eyes are just about your most precious possession. Do not neglect them. There are no substitutes for your eyes.

SIGHT-SAVING TIPS

1. The Indians wisely sought medicines from the plant kingdom for sight health. These herbs are currently available for use.

2. Herbal washes reportedly help invigorate and nourish the eyes.
3. Simple home healers for eye relaxation include tea bag applications, hot cloths, easy water washing and relaxation-exercises.

12

How to Let Nature
Rejuvenate Your Glands
for More Vital Living

Clark S. felt that the best years of his life were behind him. While still a young 44 (age is a condition of *natural* health rather than calendar years), he was given to feelings of early fatigue, sallow complexion, chronic sniffles, and a stooped position that gave him the look of an elderly man. Small wonder that Clark S. was replaced at his job. He looked old in an environment that emphasized a "Forward" and "Think Young" attitude.

He had made up his mind that it was too late to start all over again and took another job at a lower salary. Clark did not realize that his feeling of premature tiredness and his unhealthy appearance could be due to a sluggish glandular condition. Only when a co-worker was given a coveted promotion, even though he was much older (but felt much younger) than Clark, did he decide to do something.

He was told about a traditional, folk-healing elixir. It called for using selected herbs in single form or in combination, as a means of helping to put stimulating action into the gland-hormonal system, to pep up lazy organs, to stimulate them into sending forth a rich supply of nourishing "internal food." Clark tried herbs and was able to revitalize his thinking processes and soon was able to compete with others. In addition, Clark went on a program of special self-oxygenation exercises, upon being told that the hormonal system requires precious "live" air for healthful living.

A well-rounded program, that included natural and chemically untreated foods, helped put Clark S. back in the mainstream of life. It was all in his glands! The following are some of the secrets he used in stimulating his glands:

HERBAL YOUTH ELIXIR   The ancients, notably the Chinese, were aware that herbs could feed the gland-hormonal system by helping to create a natural invigoration. (Although they could not name the scientific parts, they were ahead of us in knowing how to stimulate a natural flow through natural means.) Oriental herbalists would prepare a Herbal Youth Elixir and offer it to members of the Imperial Court. Small wonder they were awarded positions of the nobility. (This Herbal Youth Elixir is based upon reported remedies of the Chinese-Tibetan healers who were credited with having the secrets of "eternal" youth and life.)

Take one ounce of each: poke root (use green root when possible), bayberry bark, white oak bark, scullcap, black cohosh. Steep in one pint of water for thirty minutes. Strain, and sip slowly. It was reported that a cupful of this elixir taken daily would produce beneficial tonic results.

HOW GYPSIES WOULD USE HERBS FOR VIGOR

The nomad gypsies of Mid-Europe had to rely almost entirely upon the forces of Nature for survival and for life itself. They discovered that several herbs, when brewed together to make a tangy potion, would help revitalize the circulatory system and provide a natural feeling of vim for the glandular-hormonal chain. This remedial herb tonic served to nourish the glands, regulate the manufacture of hormones, put invigorating pep into the circulatory system. The gypsies perpetuated this formula by word of mouth. Eventually, some outsiders who were amazed at the rejuvenation-sustaining powers of the gypsies, managed to learn the secret.

CIRCULATION PEP TONIC   Based upon folklore writings, the gypsies would take one cup of this special herbal tonic, about an hour before each meal: Steep one heaping teaspoonful of just *one* of the following herbs: Gentian root, scullcap, colombo, rue, valerian, vervain, peppermint, spearmint. Strain off and drink when comfortably hot.

Gypsies Travelled with Herbal Powders

The unusual stamina of the gypsies may be traced to their faith in these herbal powders which went with them wherever they travelled. They knew that the key to a well-nourished system that bubbles with vital living is in an improved circulation. They relied upon the woods, the forests, and the trees of Nature. These were rich sources of healing grasses and natural "gland stimulants" that helped put a natural feeling of overall youthful exuberance into their glandular system.

YOGA SECRETS OF IMPROVED GLANDULAR REJUVENATION

The mysteries of yoga are slowly becoming known to the western world. In particular, one form is known as *Raja Yoga*, a science that was known and practiced some thousands of years ago in primitive India. It involves proper meditation-breathing which reportedly will help nourish and invigorate the delicate glandular balance.

Raja Yoga uses the principle that when proper breathing exercises are performed in combination with relaxation, the glandular system will respond by an organization of always available healing forces.

Oxygen bearing nutrients thus reach the vital seven important endocrine glands; from the head downward, these are the pituitary, thyroid, parathyroids, thymus, adrenals, islet cells of the pancreas and gonads. Raja Yoga helps nourish the hormones because the oxygen is food to the internal rivers of life. Nearly all bodily activities are regulated by these glands; their hormones do not pass through tubes or ducts but pour out directly into the bloodstream. This calls for "feeding" through the bloodstream and this red river of internal life needs oxygen. The meditating Yoga devotees of India and Tibet were wise in knowing how to provide such food to the hormonal system.

Four Raja Yoga Exercises for Glandular Goodness

Here are four types of surprisingly easy Raja Yoga-based exercises that send a stream of rich oxygen to nourish your glands:

1. DOG PANTING   Ever watch a dog pant heavily? Do it the same way for 30 seconds to one minute. But don't overdo. If you feel dizziness (hyperventilation), it means too much carbon dioxide is being washed out of the blood because of increased respirations. The Raja Yoga followers of India and Tibet will just stop and go easy after a few minutes of rest.

2. STOMACH LIFT   You may do this in the home, office, or when taking a shower. Stand straight. Blow out all your air. Now bend over slightly. Keep your knees straight. Put your palms on your upper thighs. Breathe in deeply. Suck in your stomach high into your chest. Hold until you must inhale. Rest. Repeat 3 times daily. This particular Raja Yoga Rejuvenation Motion helps strengthen the diaphragm and much-neglected chest and pectoral muscles.

3. SIP YOUR BREATH   The Tibetans were wise in knowing how to "feed" their glands. They would follow this simple Raja Yoga motion: Pucker your lips as if about to whistle or drink through a straw. Now, slowly sip in the air as if your lungs were bottomless. Feel that cooling reaction? It goes all the way down to your diaphragm. Make this inhalation last as long as possible by sipping *very slowly*. Hold your breath for as long as it took you to sip in the air. Then exhale slowly. Do.this twice daily.

4. TIBETAN LAMA QUICK BELLOWS BREATH   A few chosen visitors to Tibet reported that the lamas and holy men would help revitalize their insides and restore a feeling of youth by means of this "quick bellows" motion. *To perform:* Breathe in speedily and deeply. Fill your lower lungs. Now, in the manner of a bellows, vigorously expel the breath through your mouth while simultaneously contracting your stomach muscles. This particular Tibetan Lama Quick Bellows Breath sends a fresh stream of nutrient-carrying oxygen to your bloodstream and thereby feeds your glandular system; do it modestly to avoid hyper-ventilation. At first, the experts do it just twice daily. Gradually, as they experience revitalization, they increase to ten times daily.

THE FOOD THAT AWAKENS LAZY GLANDS

Rose B. scoffed at the thought that something was "wrong" with her glands. Yet, she consented to try *alfalfa tea*. She replaced her caffeine-containing coffee and the tannic-acid containing tea with this natural herb brew. In addition, she gave up her starched and sweetened foods, nourished her system with lots of fresh fruits and vegetables. But always, alfalfa tea was her beverage with meals and whenever she felt the need for a "lift."

Alfalfa Tea Helps Awaken Lazy Glands

Rose B. soon felt more natural energy; no longer did she lie in bed in the morning, groggy and dizzy and unable to arouse herself to get out and make breakfast. Alfalfa tea helped nourish Rose B.'s hormonal channels and stimulated her lazy glands.

Benefits of Alfalfa

This healing grass has been known for several thousand years. It is said that the Arabs would use it as an elixir for their horses, claiming that the animals would become strong and fleet-footed on the desert sands. It is a prime source of hormone-feeding protein; it is also rich in the glandular cell restorative minerals such as phosphorus, iron, chlorine, potassium, silicon, magnesium. In particular, alfalfa has a prime source of calcium which provides stabilization to the nerve roots and helps create a normalization of bodily and glandular functions. All this in the simple yet powerful alfalfa.

Alfalfa in Salads and Teas

Alfalfa leaves and branches may be used for a raw vegetable salad. You may also use alfalfa seeds for steeping tea. Many health food stores sell alfalfa in tea bags for speedy use.

EARLY BIRD SELF-STARTER TONIC

Folks in the regions of Vermont (the longevity of these people is amazing!) have always relied upon natural foods for overall health. Since the emotional-physical balance is delicately maintained by a healthy set of glands, it is essential to nourish these energy producers in the morning. Most of the folks in the snow-covered hill country of Vermont are able to awaken early and start out with natural energy because of a folk tonic that is all-natural. It is traditional with many Vermonters to start off the day with this *Early Bird Self-Starter Tonic*:

Mix two tablespoons of apple cider vinegar with one cup of

freshly poured tap water. Sweeten with one teaspoon of natural organic honey. Stir vigorously, or use a blender for thorough assimilation. Drink slowly before breakfast.

Benefits of Early Bird Self-Starter Tonic

The apple cider vinegar is one of Nature's most generous sources of potassium, a mineral that helps maintain a hormonal balance in the bloodstream. Potassium is needed by the body to assist in the transportation of oxygen to the brain cells. To dispose of fatigue causing ingredients, the kidneys rely upon the glands which need potassium for invigoration and contractions. Potassium is found in abundance in apple cider vinegar and it may be this "secret" that makes this healthful tonic so beneficial to the hormones and also invigorate the long-living Vermonters.

Refresh Your Glands and Enjoy Youthful Life

Healthful oxygen-bearing exercise, nourishing food, herbal healers from the meadows and folk remedial tonics aid in refreshing the glands to put youth back into life!

PEPPY POINTS IN CHAPTER 12

1. The Herbal Youth Elixir, taken from the Chinese-Tibetan folklore, reportedly nourishes the glands and facilitates healthful hormonal function.
2. Gypsies reportedly derived superior powers and vigor through a Circulation Pep Tonic which was said to invigorate the glands.
3. Raja Yoga has been known for thousands of years as a key to hormonal happiness.
4. For happy glands, Alfalfa Tea is a tasty and easy way to nourish yourself with minerals.
5. Vermonters attribute longevity to peppy glands by means of ingredients in Early Bird Self-Starter Tonic.

13

How to Wash Your Bloodstream
for the Sparkle of
a More Youthful Life

Deep in the mountains of Switzerland, nestled in the healthful passes and clearings, are many sanatoriums and rest homes. For decades, such natural healing institutions as Dr. Rollier's, the Bircher-Benner Sanatorium and others, have devoted their efforts to healing the whole person, rather than just the specific condition complained of. In particular, these healing havens have practiced what Father Kneipp, a famous natural healer, once called "blood washing."

They learned that the bloodstream is often a polluated internal river; it becomes burdened with toxic substances, acid wastes, accumulated debris, and clogged up with scummy substances. Since the blood is the carrier of life-giving nutrients and oxygen to all parts of the body, its sparkling cleanliness is recognized as being a potent source of strength, zest and overall vitality.

HOW EUROPEAN HEALERS USE
BLOOD WASHING TECHNIQUES

To these healing havens, many of the high and the lowly of the world have appeared for help with their health. Royalty and commonfolk have all been received and healed of bodily disturbances when blood washing was used as the basis of health restoration. Self-cleaning of the bloodstream is based upon these natural programs:

133

1. CONTROLLED RAW JUICE FASTING   For upwards of one
day to one week, the person puts himself on a raw juice fast. Fresh
raw fruit and/or vegetable juices are consumed. The rich store
of vitamins and minerals in juices thereby act as a "scrubbing"
to the bloodstream and serve to wash out the accumulated debris.

2. PROPER VENTILATION FOR AERATION   Through the pores
of the skin, offensive wastes have to be given off. This requires
an "air bath" which is done by wearing loose-fitting clothes,
allowing for exposure to soothing sunshine and fresh air such as
in the mountains or on the beaches.

3. ELIMINATION OF TOXIC-CAUSING COFFEE AND TEA
These are acid-forming foods that deposit a dirty sheen on the
delicate cells and corpuscles of the bloodstream. The Swiss mountain healers require their patients to eliminate these unnatural
foods. Instead, they substitute herbal teas.

4. A HAPPY MIND CREATES HAPPY BLOOD!   Tensions,
overwork, worry, fear, anger, unhappiness and plain old-fashioned
hate greatly hinder the circulation of the blood. Thus, the impurities are not carried off as they should be. The stagnated
condition of the skin is one cause of impure blood. Swiss healers
urge their patients to have a happy mind as a means of having
happy blood!

5. CORRECT BOWEL REGULATION   Sparkling vitality begins
with regularity. Swiss healers have long used natural herbal laxatives. One popular folklore regularity herbal tonic is regarded as
most beneficial: mix thoroughly one tablespoonful each of mandrake, buckthorn bark, rhubarb root, fennel seed and calamus
root and one teaspoonful of aloes. Take one-half teaspoonful with
a glass of cold water, after meals or upon retiring.

6. THE SWISS HERB FOR INTERNAL REGULARITY   The Swiss
healers maintain firmly that toxic wastes in the bloodstream can
be washed out by the use of mandrake. They take one-fourth
teaspoonful of powdered *mandrake* in a half glass of cold water,
followed by a glass of hot water. They prefer this to be done before
retiring.

7. THE SWISS BLOOD WASHING COCKTAIL   Natives swear
by this herbal-based cocktail: mix thoroughly one ounce mandrake
root, one ounce cascara sagrada bark, one ounce buckthorn bark,
one ounce fennel seed, one ounce calamus root and one-fourth

ounce aloes. Mix thoroughly by putting through a fine sieve. (Modern herbalists have them in powdered form.) Take one-half teaspoonful with a glass of hot water upon retiring. Helps soothe the digestive system and also acts as a "magnet" in sucking up the accumulated wastes and cellular trash that infest the bloodstream.

HOW HELEN J. RELIEVED HER "TIRED BLOOD"

Helen J. should have been in the prime of her life, except that the bloom in her cheeks was gone. She complained that she had "tired blood" because she felt worn out and sick all the time. Improper blood flow as well as poor cleansing had led to the formation of sluggish wastes.

Helen J. was given a program of iron-feeding for the blood. (Iron is a mineral that helps repair and replenish the cells of the bloodstream. Iron is found in apricots, raisins, liver, molasses, egg yolk, green vegetables and nuts.) Helen J. did not like the taste of liver so she took desiccated liver capsules which are sold at most health food shops and vitamin outlets. (Desiccated liver is a capsule product that has all the blood washing nutrients in liver but without its connective tissue and fat.) After a while, in addition to a program of natural, healthful food, Helen J. experienced revitalized living.

But she became too overly confident; Helen J. reverted back to poor diet and discontinued her blood washing by means of iron-rich foods. She soon developed serious anemia which required hospitalization.

THE FOOD THAT HELPS WASH THE BLOODSTREAM

The golden apricot has long been hailed as a prime source of iron and copper and a host of precious minerals that are needed for washing the bloodstream. The nutrients in the golden apricot contain elements that appear in the oxygen-carrying hemoglobin fraction of the red blood cells. Apricot juice has long been favored by Swiss healers and many in other natural healing institutions. They recognized that apricot juice is a prime source of the basic nutrients that nourish the hemoglobin and is responsible for the transport of oxygen from the lungs to the other body cells. In some of the Swiss or Bavarian mountain sanatoriums, the healers put their patients on a raw apricot juice fast for several days as a means of initiating this blood cleaning action. This puts the patients on the road to blood washed good health.

SALT RUB OPENS PORES TO PERMIT VENTILATION

Bruce E. takes an early morning bath, then he helps open his pores by a time-tested folk tip known as the Salt Rub. He thoroughly massages himself with ordinary coarse salt. Then he sprinkles himself with a needle-spray shower and he feels great with that good-to-be-alive sensation that denotes healthy blood. The benefit here is that the abrasive and coarse friction of the salt helps open the clogged pores to permit infectious gaseous wastes to come out and be cast off. Bruce E. not only feels better, but he looks younger, too.

WATER: KEY TO CLEAN BLOOD

Drinking fresh water is Nature's key to clean and washed blood. Many healers have urged that a daily schedule of six to eight glasses of water be included in the blood washing program.

Benefits of Water Drinking

Circulation Is Supercharged. When taken into the stomach and intestinal canal, water is received into the blood and increases its volume. Then fullness of the circulatory vessels is increased. They are never expanded to their fullest extent. This fullness-increase permits room for a change in the volume of their contents. Water drinking makes the blood more fluid and circulation is quickened by its dilution.

Water Helps Wash Off Wastes. Water causes a natural waste washing through the lungs, skin, kidneys, intestines. Water has a remarkable dissolving action; the poisons that are separated from the tissues are dissolved. Then the volume of the blood is increased; more water helps wash off waste matter in every part, thereby facilitating in removal. This is seen by increased waste secretions and perspiration.

Water Improves Resistance to Colds. Water helps in the washing and rebuilding of tissues. Correct water drinking helps activate skin function and thereby increase the circulation which, in turn, builds resistance to colds and allergic tendencies.

Water Improves Circulation. About 90% of blood plasma is

water. This liquidity allows blood plasma to circulate freely throughout the body, carrying vital substances with it. Among these substances are food, gases, inorganic salts, waste products. Water is needed to help plasma circulation and to carry discarded sludge into the secretory organs such as the liver, kidneys, sweat glands and digestive glands. A washed bloodstream also carries carbon dioxide to the lungs to be given off.

Self-Test for Blood Cleanliness

It has been noted that when the body's urine is acid, then the blood is comparatively clean because of its water supply. You can test any possible water deficiency, with your doctor's approval, by this simple method:

Go to any pharmacy and purchase Squibb-Nitrazine paper. Dip a small corner of this paper in your urine sample. A chart on the nitrazine paper container will provide more explicit instructions; or, ask your physician. If the paper is yellow, your blood has reasonable cleanliness: If the paper is another color, it means your urine is too alkaline and you need to wash your blood with natural fresh juices and lots of water drinking.

Plain Water Helps Wash Bloodstream

Water is an essential constituent of living protoplasm. No cell functions when it is absolutely dry, and most cells must be constantly bathed in fluid in order to help keep clean. Waste-bearing water (urine) is necessary to flush away the end products of metabolism. Without water, the bloodstream becomes clogged as a sludged pond and is a site for infectious reactions. Plain water is the answer to a healthy bloodstream.

Contrast Applications Help Relieve Blood Congestion

Natural blood washing healers often reported success with contrast applications of cold and hot water. These were applied to the parts that were insufficiently blood nourished. Clogged blood pockets choked off a flow of nourishment to these other parts. By applying comfortably hot poultices or clothes to a "cold" or "aching" part, the warmth helps to magnetically draw blood to its "starved" region and thus provide relief.

Healing Benefits of Water

Water is an essential constituent of tissue cells and all body fluids, such as the bloodstream. Water also helps dissolve nutritive material in the course of digestion, so that it can be absorbed into the blood, which carries it to various parts of the body for repairing and then for removal as waste. Water also keeps all the mucous membranes of the body soft and prevents friction of their surface. Water may be regarded Nature's perfect blood washer. It helps dissolve poisonous waste materials and foreign elements in the bloodstream, thereby aiding their elimination. Its *diaphoretic* action is a form of cleansing because it induces perspiration. This helps slough off much of the infectious sludge and mucus.

SPARKLING HEALTH BEGINS WITH WASHED BLOOD

The Swiss and mountain healers long realized that Nature's herbs, fresh fruits and vegetables, mineral-rich waters helped restore health through a sparkling bloodstream . . . the river of life!

MAIN POINTS OF CHAPTER 13

1. A clean bloodstream helps build health; Swiss healers recognized the values of raw juice fasting, proper ventilation, emotional stability, herbal cleansing for washing the bloodstream.
2. Internal regularity often requires a Swiss-inspired herbal self-cleanser. Mandrake is such a self-cleansing herb.
3. The Swiss use a Blood Washing Cocktail to help suck up accumulated wastes and cellular trash that cause infections to the bloodstream.
4. Tired blood becomes alert through iron and apricots.
5. Wash away clogged pores with a Salt Rub.
6. Water is Nature's antiseptic cleanser for the bloodstream.

14

A Slenderizing Program
to "Trim and Stay Trim"

Elsa N. loved to eat. She could not resist double portions at mealtime; neither could she resist those calorie-rich salad dressings as well as juicy good desserts. Elsa N. was so bulky that when she attended a social affair with her husband, someone erroneously thought that Elsa was his mother! Overweight certainly made her look much older and it was this innocent mistake that started her dieting.

HOW TO EAT AND SLIM DOWN

Elsa N. found hundreds, even thousands, who loved to eat when she attended a special seminar held under the guidance and auspices of a large city's team of doctors. This doctor-team prepared a special set of easy-to-follow eating plans that enabled the "fatties" to eat while they slimmed down. This was the answer to their food-loving dreams. Elsa N. followed this "Trim and Stay Trim" eating program and shed so many pounds that she was later happily mistaken for her husband's younger sister! Here is the simple program that enables overweights to have their cake and eat it, too!

TASTY FOODS TO BECOME TRIM-SLIM

1. You may follow this program unless there is a medical reason for not reducing. You will need to follow your physician's advice.
2. You may drink water freely.
3. You may have tea or coffee, using some of your fat-free milk

if desired. *Use no sugar.* Saccharin or similar sweeteners may be substituted.

4. You may use beef or chicken broth after the fat has been skimmed off, or you may use bouillon cubes for clear soup.

5. You may use lemon juice or vinegar or tomato juice for salad dressings.

6. You may use seasonings such as salt (unless on low sodium diet), pepper, paprika, garlic, herbs, celery seeds, mustard or vinegar.

7. Meat, fish and poultry should be broiled, pan-broiled, boiled, baked or roasted, without added fat. NEVER FRIED. Remove all visible fat before eating. Do not eat gravies or sauces.

8. Eggs should be cooked in the shell or poached.

9. Vegetables may be eaten raw or cooked without fat or sauces or salad oil dressings.

10. Fruits may be eaten raw or cooked without sugar. If fruit canned in syrup is used, rinse off syrup with hot water and chill.

11. Your diet should include two cups of fat-free milk or fat-free buttermilk. You may use this to suit your desires. You may use some of it in tea or coffee; or drink it at mealtime or in-between meals or at bedtime.

12. EAT ALL YOU WANT of the following vegetables, raw or cooked, without added fat, sauces or oil dressings. Any of them may be eaten between meals if you are hungry:

asparagus	mung bean sprouts
beet greens	mushrooms
broccoli	mustard greens
cabbage	parsley
cauliflower	peppers
celery	pickles, sour or dill
chard	pimientos
Chinese cabbage	radishes
collards	sauerkraut
cucumber	spinach
dandelion greens	squash, summer
endive	string beans, young
escarole	turnip greens
kale	watercress
lettuce	

13. EAT ONE PORTION DAILY of the following vegetables:

artichokes	parsnips
bamboo shoots	peas
beets	pumpkin
Brussels sprouts	rutabagas
carrots	scallions
eggplant	squash, winter
kohlrabi	string beans, mature
leeks	turnips
okra	tomato
onions	tomato juice
oyster plant	

14. DO NOT EAT OR DRINK any of the following without advice from your doctor:

alcohol beverages	lima beans
(beer, wine, whiskey)	macaroni
avocado	margarine
bacon or back fat	marmalade
butter	mayonnaise
cake	noodles
candy	nuts
Chinese food	oil
chocolate	olives
cocoanut	pancakes
cookies	peanut butter
corn (fresh or canned)	pies
crackers	plantains
doughnuts	popcorn
dried fruits	potatoes
dried peas or beans	potato chips
French dressing	pretzels
French fries	puddings
fried foods	rice
gravy	soda, gingerale, cola
honey	soybeans
ice cream; ices	spaghetti
jam	sugar & syrups
jelly	sweet & sour cream
lentils	waffles

TASTY BENEFITS OF THE
"TRIM AND STAY TRIM" PROGRAM

This highly successful program was followed by many plump and chubby people with appetizing delight. It enabled them to forget about calories; many who were compulsive eaters were deliciously pleased to eat fully, nutritionally and wholesomely of the "eat all you want" group of tasty foods. For those who almost wept at having to pass up rich dressings, the use of lemon-tomato juice was such a lip-smacking taste thrill, they declared enjoyment at having to lose weight because of the juicy good taste of such a dressing.

"Trim and Stay Trim" Program Becomes
Basis for Overweight Watching Groups

The success of this eat-and-slim-down program was so great, that several enterprising chubbies formed their own pound watchers groups and used the preceding line up as the basis for their organization. Happy slim-down folks responded to group therapy at meetings and followed the tasty do's and don'ts of the doctor-prepared program.

Puts a Curb on Runaway Appetite

Evelyn J., a plump 265-pound housewife, found this program a delicious triumph over her runaway appetite. Previously, she would gorge herself on everything and anything she could get her hands (and mouth) upon. Now, she would prepare a dish of steamed mushrooms and cauliflower, douse them with tomato juice dressing and stuff herself until her appetite eased. That was how she developed a natural self-control and was able to cut down on runaway eating.

Nick A. Reduces Paunch with Meat Eating

At first, Nick was called "Tubby" behind his back by the coworkers in the office. Then when his paunch developed another paunch, he was called "Tubby" right to his red face. His double chin and jowls burned in red-faced shame. He had tried diet drugs with serious physical reactions. He had tried exercise but his appetite became more enormous after physical exercise. Will power was not his gift. He attended the special group meetings and explained that he liked to eat meat. This does have high caloric count because of the animal fat. But Nick was able to continue eating meat, while removing ALL visible fat and shunning ALL gravies and sauces. He followed the other program suggestions and after several months, his first paunch went down. The second soon slipped off and now the name "Tubby" is out of place. Nick is a new and younger man.

"So Many Good Things to Eat While Reducing."

Freda P. loved good things to eat. She loved the Trim program but she became so enamoured with the permitted foods that she disregarded the other rules and gorged herself without limit. Even the "one portion" foods became six portions. Freda lost much of her weight but when she discontinued the program, she gained it right back again. Yes, the good things that are to be eaten all the time may be enjoyed while reducing. But the "one portion" and "no portion at all" foods as well as the special slim guidelines about cooking and preparation, must be included for reducing success. Freda became morose and unhappy in her stuffed teddy bear plumpness. She took to overeating as a means of compensating for her frustration and this made her a hopeless fatty. If only she had followed the program with faithfulness. She could have, today, been as slim as a movie star!

HOLLYWOOD'S SECRET OF APPETITE CONTROL

A noted pencil-slim film star is able to control the sometimes nagging compulsion to eat by mixing three tablespoons of apple cider vinegar in a glass of water. She stirs vigorously and drinks whenever the eating mood hits her. She is able to satisfy her appetite with this simple health cocktail.

Cucumber Juice Highball for Hunger-Taming

A fashion model, Grace B., who wants to tame the hunger urge, sips a glass of cucumber juice. The alkaline content offers a soothing relaxation to the urge to eat and Grace B. is thus able to avoid eating between meals (the real overweight culprit). Furthermore, she will drink one glass of cucumber juice about a half hour before a meal. This helps tame her appetite and she eats modestly and healthfully. Many diet shops have prepared cucumber juice available in bottles or cans. You may squeeze the juice at home. Select organic cucumbers.

How Sauerkraut Puts the Curb on Wild Hunger

Norman F., a desk-bound fatty, was unable to follow any reducing program. There was something "wild" about his taste buds that compelled him to stuff himself throughout the day. He heard of a folk drink that would ease the urge for hunger. It consisted of ordinary sauerkraut juice (sold at most health stores and special diet shops).

Norman tried it with the happy result that his taste buds were soothed and relaxed. This eased his urge for constant eating. Now, he drinks one glass at each of the following hours: ten o'clock in the morning, two o'clock in the afternoon, four o'clock and then a final glass about an hour before his main dinner. This gives him a steady time-clock precision to offer a gradual curb on his wild hunger.

Benefits of Sauerkraut Juice

Folklore tells that the battling Vikings and the Saxons who were given to enormous feasts of victory, would have to slim down before being able to go forth in battle again. They would drink copious amounts of sauerkraut juice to calm the appetite. The secret here is that a tart-tangy taste in sauerkraut juice helps satisfy the taste buds and ease the eating compulsion. In many of the modern European health resorts, sauerkraut juice is the main beverage given to overweights.

Drinking Water Eases Appetites

Water is a nutrient, second only to oxygen in health benefit. It is reported that drinking two glasses of water *before* each meal helps keep the stomach comfortable, makes it easier to eat less, and aids in good digestion and intestinal regularity. Nature always knows best!

Fresh Fruit for Juicy Good Dessert

Delicious fruits for dessert will ease the need for the calorie-high cakes and pies which are mostly sugar and starch. Healthful slimming desserts are peaches, pears, oranges, grapefruit, watermelon, cantaloupe, cherries, seasonal berries. For an exotic touch, try some of these: Hawaiian papaya, Japanese persimmons, Crenshaw melons and Malaga, Muscat and Flame Tokay grapes.

HEALTH SECRETS FOR MELTING POUNDS WHILE EATING JOYFULLY

Long before diet was discovered, overweight folks throughout the world developed instinctive and folklore secrets for melting pounds while eating joyfully. Here are several traditional European and American health secrets:

DAIRY DELIGHTS   Use skimmed milk in cooking and for drinking; try buttermilk. Reliquified nonfat dry milk, a money and calorie saver, is tastefully slimming.

SOUR CREAM SUBSTITUTE   Whip or beat cottage cheese smooth in a blender and then use in place of sour cream.

NATURAL FRUIT SYRUP   Wherever possible, use fresh fruits. If you must use canned fruits, drain off the heavy syrup and replace with fresh fruit juice. This makes a natural "syrup" that is slimmingly delicious. You may prefer fruits sweetened with non-nutritive sweeteners.

GRAVY WITH A LIGHT TOUCH   Instead of meat drippings, make gravy with bouillon as a base. This gives it a light and slimming touch.

LOW-CALORIE APPETITE THRILLERS   Select clear broths or vegetable soups, spiced fruit or vegetable juices. Helps thrill without filling.

CASSEROLES ON A CALORIE BUDGET   Put casseroles in the refrigerator overnight; it makes it easy to skim off calorie-heavy fat that rises to the surface.

CURVACEOUS CREAM SAUCES   When sautéing foods or making cream sauces, use half the fat specified. Substitute skimmed milk, whenever it's suitable, for whole milk.

DRINK YOURSELF SLIM   Drink coffee or tea, whenever you wish to put a slimming curb on an appetite. But skip the milk, cream or sugar. Europeans prefer sipping bouillon for a slimming appetite-relaxant. Takes the edge off the eating urge.

Remember: Reducing is the test of more than just will power. It calls for satisfying a physical need and selecting slimming foods that fill without fattening. Take advantage of the wealth of folk reducers presented herein and the Trim and Stay Trim Program that was doctor-prepared and nationally accepted with slimming success!

IN SUMMARY OF THIS CHAPTER

1. The Trim-Slim Program, a doctor-prepared slimming feast, has helped countless overweights become slim while they ate with relish!
2. Hollywood's Secret of Appetite Control is now available to the public. Costs just pennies per glass.
3. Sauerkraut Juice, a Saxon slimming folklore secret, works in modern European exclusive salons.
4. Water-drinking is Nature's built in curb-control-appetite.
5. Europeans knew how to use substitutions to soothe appetite-taste and slim down.

15

How to Get
the Energy-Building Power of
Natural "Peptimism"

The founders of the corporate giants of today were usually men of enviable vitality and youthful energy. They labored long hours, under arduous conditions, yet managed to create some of the most ingenius inventions and brilliant ideas that helped build a mighty nation. All of this was done in the days when modern science was still in its infancy and energy in health was a new word to the dictionary. The early builders drew from the folksy wisdom of common sense people who were able to create self-awakening through natural means.

This chapter will draw upon past and present secrets of energy-building. It will reveal an untapped, hidden source of great vitality. It lies deep within your thought patterns, just waiting to be alerted. Once this power, known as *peptimism*, is touched off, it can help supercharge the mind and body and release a dynamic built-in vitality that can influence health, happiness and the success pattern.

What is *peptimism?* It is a source of enthusiasm and ambition that helps erase tension blocks, helps melt away unnatural fatigue, helps nourish those "lazy" ambitions that need fulfillment.

Peptimism calls for the utilization of a proper *attitude* toward the responsibilities and problems of yesterday, today and tomorrow. Once you have marshalled the built-in forces of the emotions to create a stimulating attitude, you have been able to tap the hidden source of power through peptimism. It begins with an *emotion-strengthening* program.

THE FIVE-STEP EMOTIONAL-PEPTIMISM PROGRAM

A study was made by Drs. Charles Solley and Kenneth Mumden at the Menninger Foundation; the following program was created for releasing the hidden and energy-building sources of peptimism. These forces reportedly help strengthen the emotions and have been utilized by the greatest men of the past to help build a mighty nation. Here is their outlined five-step program designed to supercharge the emotions with peptimism:

1. *Develop a wide variety of sources of gratification.* You are not required to chase frenetically from one activity to another, but rather, to seek pleasure in many different ways and from many things. If, for any reason, you should lose one source of gratification, then you can turn to another, or still another. Peptimism is energized into revitalizing your being when you are able to find interest and emotional rapport in a variety of different fields.

2. *Become flexible when you face stress and tension.* Peptimism calls for being able to roll with the punches. When faced with problems, seek an alternative solution, do not become part of the problem. Flexibility under stress is closely related to having a wide variety of sources of gratification. Rather than buck the wind, find ways to shield yourself and also a way out of the problem. With more supports to fall back upon, you will be less threatened by situations that produce fear and anxiety. By "bending with the wind," you will muster your built-in forces of peptimism and be able to face problems with courage and conviction.

3. *Recognize and accept your limitations as well as your assets.* Peptimism is unleashed and goes to work to nourish the emotional powers when you admit that you have both limitations as well as assets. One of the old-time folk suggestions is: *develop an accurate picture of yourself.* Take pride in what you see. You need not be smug and complacent about yourself, but know that you are an individual with certain abilities that will be used to the utmost—no more! Do the best you can and strive to be a leader in your chosen work.

4. *Treat others as individuals.* You will be energizing pepti-

mism when you really *care* about what other people feel. If you are overly preoccupied with yourself and if you erroneously pay only superficial attention to others, then you will be locking away the power of peptimism. Unleash it with care and kindness for others and help enrich yourself, in return.

5. *Peptimism calls for being active and productive.* Use your powers in your own behalf and in behalf of others. Do what you do because you like to do it and you enjoy using your skills. You should not feel driven to produce to prove yourself. Rather, seek achievement for what you can *do,* not for what you can *be*; for when you try to *be* something or someone, you may never be satisfied with yourself even if you achieve the desired goal. Peptimism reaches its height when you *do* something and with the doing, you become someone!

Your lifespan is to be lived. If you have good emotional health, live life to the fullest; if you live life enjoyably, you will be endowing yourself with the basics of good emotional health. This releases the hidden powers of peptimism.

DIPLOMACY UNLEASHES PEPTIMISM

Nearly everyone tells you to be diplomatic about this thing or that thing, but few will tell you how—and few will tell you the benefits of being diplomatic! Let's draw upon the secrets of some of the greatest diplomats of the past and see how it can work to release peptimism to help enrich lives in many ways.

Visible Diplomacy

Peptimism is unleased when you are diplomatic by developing *patience.* In a word: *wait!* Bide your time! Things will work out when you use leisurely thought.

Hurry Can Be Self-Defeating

As soon as you try to unnecessarily hurry a situation along, you take the reins away and you can defeat your program. Go slow and steady; even if it is unusually slow, take note that it is moving and that it will be reasonably error-free. This is a key to diplomacy and peptimism. Else, you drain yourself out and vitality is gone.

Peptimism Is Cautious and Progressive

Peptimism calls for you to take your time, realizing that patience is the key to diplomatic success, that the slow pace at which you are traveling now is really the fastest time in which the task can be consummated; all intermediate delays, discouragements, distractions, or setbacks are stepping stones to your final success. The slightest surrender to impatience on your part represses your power of peptimism. Be patient and your diplomacy will unleash the success-building power of peptimism.

SELF-ENERGIZING RELEASES POWER OF PEPTIMISM

It is often maintained that more than half of the population "live dull, routine lives." This was not so in the past when folks took pride and satisfaction in their projects. You need to ask yourself if a dull, routine life applies to you. By means of developing peptimism which is a combination of energy-enthusiasm, routine and dullness tend to evaporate.

Release Resentments and Self-Rejuvenate

Clyde A. went to his doctor for treatment of chronic fatigue. He was in good physical health, yet he was constantly tired; he complained that life was dull and boring. The doctor told him, "Your trouble is your built-up supply of resentments. They're like poisons. They burn away your source of vitality and energy. What I suggest you do is talk it out to a psychiatrist, clergyman or any other sympathetic soul. Get rid of your anxieties and resentments, talk out your guilt feelings and discouragements. That helps self-cleanse your mind and you'll replace these fatigue-poisons with healthful peptimism."

Clyde A. followed this advice and was soon "light as air" and happy. He had cast off negatives and now replaced them with positives. Once this was done, peptimism was unleashed. He became imbued with excitement about God, life, people, his family, opportunities. He developed peptimism-enthusiasm for his daily tasks and now he enjoyed his job. He earned more money. The success pattern was established by marshalling and releasing the forces of peptimism!

LIVE OUTSIDE YOURSELF VIA PEPTIMISM

We know about the difference between introverts and extroverts. One will live within himself and the other is more gregarious and will live outside of himself. You can improve your personality. It is not inherited. You may inherit your anatomical "chassis" but your disposition is up to you. Peptimism is within all of us. It is up to your own personal thinking patterns to release this treasure of success and energy. Many of the greatest builders of the world have utilized peptimism and have based success on some of these working suggestions:

Create a Compliment Club with One Member—Yourself

That's the key to unlocking peptimism. Create your own Compliment Club with yourself as the only member. Turn your attention off yourself and focus on others around you. Look for their merits or virtues and offer them a sincere bit of praise. Set a goal: compliment three different people each day. Note how they accept your praise. It makes them feel good. It makes you feel good. Where does that good feeling come from? You guessed it— the built-in supply of natural peptimism. You released it by complimenting.

Turn Off Your Introverted Clock and Set Off an Extroverted Clock

Picture yourself as an alarm clock. The introverted clock is hardly heard and is too self-wrapped. The extroverted clock is a loud and noticeable alarm. Become that "alarm" by thinking of others rather than yourself. Once you have done this, you release your peptimism-source and benefits become available.

YOUR EMOTIONAL SELF-OILING PROGRAM

To make the most of peptimism, check your emotional self-oil. You will want to avoid a burned-out bearing. The oil of human relationships is a precious built-in fluid stemming from peptimism. Keep it at a proper level so it helps you get the most that life has to offer. Here is a simple program for emotional self-oiling that helps peptimism work smoothly and without friction or rust:

1. When you talk to another person, try to understand his thought processes and motives so you will understand *why* he says *what* he says. Guide and suggest, but do not contradict or scold.

2. Banish from thought any remarks that cut or hurt or sting. If you are unable to say anything kind, say nothing!

3. Seek out the good, the bright, the cheerful. Oh, you will find much blight and disappointment but rather than obsess your thoughts with this negative attitude, seek the good and the hopeful. The unpleasant things in life, from the little, everyday disappointments to the big things that may seem to crush us, are always (not sometimes, but always) experiences that contain good. Such experiences are not tragedies or defeats that we are "fated" to undergo, nor are they trials that are sent to test us. Instead, they are opportunities for us to move us a step in emotional health. Move up more and more steps and when you reach the desired height, you will have reaped the wondrous benefits of peptimism.

4. Here is a professional clinician's way of easing tension and helping to release emotional powers of peptimism:

Sit in a straight chair with both feet flat on the floor. Let your hands rest relaxed in your lap, with your shoulders sagging forward. Close your eyes and let your head hang loose in front of your chest. Relax as completely as possible, part by part. Continue deliberate relaxation until you cannot feel stiffness or tension anywhere in your body. This usually takes about one minute. Then lift your right hand to shoulder height and let it fall limply into your lap again. Do the same with your left hand. Try to relax part by part even more completely. After another minute, you will find that you are able to take up the cares of the day in a much more relaxed and comfortable way.

Benefits of Above Tension-Easer

Reportedly, the benefits include a boosted efficiency and mental calm that enabled businessmen and housewives to self-rejuvenate. It was suggested that one such Tension-Easer per hour helps marshal and stir up the built-in forces of peptimism. This is based upon an ancient form of Yoga that has been rediscovered and is now helping many people throughout the world. Much stems from the released power of peptimism that is like a hidden treasure awaiting discovery.

SUMMARY OF THIS CHAPTER

1. Peptimism is a hidden source of emotional vitality that is released through proper attitudes and kindness toward others.
2. Live outside yourself and help enrich attitudes and the potential of health, happiness and success.
3. An emotional self-oiling program helps create popularity and happiness.
4. Clinicians have reported success with the Tension-Easer that takes moments per day and adds life to your years!

16

How to
Look and Feel Younger
with Naturally Dynamic Digestive Power

Folklore healings, taken from the hills of the Ozarks and the mountains of the so-called hillbilly area, reportedly provided soothing comfort to a rebellious digestion. Herbal medicines, grain-made potions, and traditional elixirs were known to these hill folk who lived in the mountains, isolated from mass-produced medicines and chemical drugs. These hardy mountain folk tilled the soil, carved out villages and cities, and enjoyed healthfully long and useful lives. They swore by traditional natural healers and would casually refer to "Granny's" homemade health tonic that reportedly put "youth" into the digestive system and made one feel fit as a mountaineer's fiddle!

GRANNY'S TUMMY TONIC   One time-honored folk healer is known as Granny's Tummy Tonic. It reportedly puts vitality into the digestive system so that the entire person enjoys youthful health. Hill folks would make it out of these ingredients, that can be bought at your local health food store:

Take 2 cups of whole grain bran, 1 cup whole grain oatmeal and mix with 4 quarts of water. Let soak overnight. In the morning, beat with an egg beater; strain through a fine sieve. Season with vegetized salt, if desired. Sip slowly in the morning to awaken a sluggish stomach.

Why Granny's Tummy Tonic Is a Digestion-Booster

The secret natural powerhouse in this all-natural tonic is *iron*. This mineral owes its unique digestion-helping role, in body metabolism, to other substances. Thus, the iron-containing hemoglobin in red blood cells can take on extra oxygen when the blood circulates through the lungs, can carry this oxygen to the enzyme-digestive tissues and there pass it to the tissue cells for oxidative processes necessary to life. As hemoglobin gives up oxygen to the tissues, it takes on carbon dioxide, a waste product of tissues, for transport to the lungs to exchange for oxygen, and the life-bringing cycle continues. Granny's Tummy Tonic is a powerhouse of such digestion-boosting iron.

How Elimination Is Aided by Granny's Tummy Tonic

Mountain folk knew nothing of commercially prepared laxatives; they probably never needed any because this traditional Tonic favored a natural regularity. Bran is composed largely of cellulose which, when prepared in the Tonic form, provides natural bulk for normal laxation. Small wonder that Granny's Tummy Tonic was a complete folk healer for the digestive tract of the hill people.

How Louisa R. Awakened Her Lazy Digestion

No matter how carefully she prepared her meals, Louisa R. suffered recurring gall bladder and digestive distress. She had gas cramps, bloating and belching. She met with a relative who had just returned from a trip to Europe. The relative said that many Europeans were able to eat hot, spicy and somewhat volatile foods with little aftereffects. Their secret? Many relied upon an old Spanish-Italian folk healer: They would take two or three tablespoonfuls of olive oil *before* each meal. The reported benefit here is that the olive oil starts a soothing flow of bile from the gall bladder, before the rest of the food enters the stomach. This helped awaken a lazy digestion and permitted improvement. Louisa R. tried it and experienced a youthful digestive system. Now she can eat heartily with little aftereffects.

HERBS FOR A HAPPY STOMACH

Long time herbalists have recommended the use of natural medicines from the woods and forests for helping to soothe frazzled digestive systems. Taken from folklore herbal writings, these appear to be the reported medicine-grasses that would help pour balm over the troubled waters of the stomach:

Take one-fourth teaspoon of any *one* of the following herbs, with a glass of water, upon arising: angelica, thyme, valerian, vervain, wild cherry, camomile, marjoram, comfrey, fennel, origanum (herb reportedly soothes sour stomach), plantain, rue, cedron.

MORNING PEP-UP HERB TONIC   Ralph was a businessman who had a nervous stomach. He became addicted to "fizz" powders and bubbly concoctions that served to make him all the more sensitive. Ralph took a trip to the South and chanced upon traditional herb tonics taken in the morning. At a hotel where he stayed, a fellow businessman told him that he would drink this natural Morning Pep-Up Herb Tonic and feel all right for the rest of the day:

Upon arising, drink one-fourth teaspoon of golden seal in a glass of piping hot water, before taking anything else in the stomach.

Ralph tried it and experienced some relief. But he became impatient with the slow recovery and went back to the patent medicines that offered "instant" relief but no cure. If he had remained with Nature, he might have enjoyed a youthful stomach.

THE HERB THAT WORKS WHILE YOU SLEEP   In the mountain country, everyone swears to the power of a delicious tea. It is made from *red raspberry* (available in powder form at most herbalists or health stores) and it is taken about two hours before going to sleep. The rich Vitamin C and the remedial antiseptic qualities go to work while you sleep. By morning, they have helped soothe and heal frazzled enzymes and a happy stomach is a happy morning! Red raspberry tea is Nature's own nightcap! The mountain folk have a traditional saying, "Red raspberry tea tonight, tomorrow all right."

HERBS FOR METABOLISM MAGIC

The key to youthful and vibrant digestion is in metabolism; this is a natural process that transforms ingested food into valuable nutrients that serve to build and sustain all body functions. A sluggish metabolism is a sluggish digestion which, in turn, is a sluggish person. *You are what you assimilate, not necessarily what you eat.*

Time-tested healing medicines from Nature in the form of herbs have long been used by those who sought a drugless way to invigorate, awaken and supercharge metabolism.

METABOLISM MAGIC HERBS   Mix equal parts golden seal, echinacea, burnet, wood betony, myrrh and spearmint. Use powdered herbs. After thoroughly mixing these together, take one-half teaspoonful in a glass of hot water one hour before meals and one upon retiring. Again we see how herbs work while you sleep! Natural "forest medicines" in these herbs help soothe and invigorate the digestive system and metabolic processes. These are the keys to golden health!

RAW FRUIT JUICE FAST   The ancients who suffered from overeating would go on a raw fruit juice fast as a means of helping to replenish their overworked digestive glands. Today, modern health salons and those traditional health resorts have taken a tip from the ancients. They, too, put their tummy-tortured guests on a raw juice fast. To follow: for one or two days, take no food except fresh raw fruit juices. The benefit here is that the overworked digestive system is given a chance to rest so that the enzymes will be strong enough to later digest incoming food.

FRUIT SOUP FOR STOMACH TONE-UP   Around the turn of the century, digestion was treated with a delicious fruit soup. Grandmother, who would squeeze into a whale-bone corset and had stomach troubles of her own, would swear by this Fruit Soup which had been handed down by her own Granny. Here's how to make it:

Take 2 cups raisins, 2 cups prunes and put in 4 quarts cold water. Let simmer until done (it would be good to first soak them overnight in the water, then they will need very little cooking). Add 1 cup unsweetened grape juice and 2 lemons, peeled and sliced very thin. Sweeten with honey to taste. May be served piping hot or cold. The rich supply of vitamins and minerals in this Fruit Soup reportedly provided blessed happiness to an overtaxed metabolism.

HOME TONICS FOR GAS RELIEF

The embarrassment of stomach gas is also unhealthy; it is a sign of indigestion; food has become fermented and created a sour stomach. While the folks who depend upon mountain healing were not well versed in medical terminology, they relied upon traditional herbs and grasses as forest medicines. They looked to the healing herbs for relief of stomach gas.

MINT TEA FOR SOOTHING STOMACH   Peppermint and spearmint tea are regarded as soothing to help ease stomach gas. Herbalists suggest equal parts of calamus root, valerian with peppermint, granulated. Mix together. Use one teaspoonful to a cup of boiling water. Steep, strain and drink one half cupful an hour *before* meals and another half cupful an hour *after* meals. The above herbs can be used in powdered form, as well as in capsules, if preferred.

STOMACH CLEANSING HERBS   The early pioneers realized that strong digestion begins with a clean stomach. One time-honored Stomach Cleaning Herbal Elixir was this one: Take one-fourth teaspoonful powdered golden seal in one-half glass of piping hot water an hour before each meal.

SUPER-PLUS STOMACH PEP-UP   In one pint of boiling water, put one heaping teaspoonful golden seal, one-fourth teaspoonful myrrh. Steep. Take a swallow a few moments before a meal is begun. The rich source of ingredients that create a demulcent (soothing) effect help pep up the digestive powers and put youth into the stomach. These herbs also reportedly feature an internal emollient (soothing and softening-feeling to inflamed parts) reaction that helps create a feeling of "happiness" for the stomach.

HOW LEMONS RESTORE YOUTH TO DIGESTION

The citrus fruit, the lemon, may well be considered Nature's pale golden treasure of youth. It is a prime source of cellular building Vitamin C; furthermore, lemons contain potassium which nourishes the nerve cells (nervous stomach may respond to lemon healing), and they are a good source of calcium and magnesium to help form albumen in the bloodstream. This ingredient heals frazzled digestive cells and tissues and knits them together to help create rejuvenated cellular rebuilding.

LEMON COCKTAIL FOR DIGESTION GOODNESS   Adele R. was able to help heal her nervous stomach by eating mild foods and also by beginning a meal with a Lemon Cocktail. Folks laughed at this "old wive's tale" but they became envious when they saw how her digestion become youthified over a period of time. The simple cocktail is made by squeezing the juice of a fresh lemon into one glass of tap water. Stir vigorously and sip slowly, about an hour before mealtime. Enzymes in the lemon juice help replenish tired digestive cells. Now, Adele R. can enjoy her food with the gustatory appreciation of a youngster.

METABOLISM: KEY TO YOUTHFUL HEALTH

Properly eaten food can help build vibrant health through metabolism. Assimilation requires a youthful digestive system. The folk healers were aware of this "key" to overall health and they sought out natural, folk-time remedial sources from the meadows and fields. Today, modern herbalists do a thriving business with these time-honored kitchen medicines, so to speak. Granny was far ahead of her time when she brewed old-fashioned herbal tonics in her cabin kitchen. Today, these same herbal healers are sold in containers of various types. They have helped thousands upon thousands for more decades than we care to count. It is hoped they will continue to offer blessed relief—through Nature—for many more decades to come.

SUMMARY OF THIS CHAPTER

1. Granny's Tummy Tonic reportedly eased digestive distress of hill and mountain folks.
2. Dispel morning blues with an all-natural Morning Pep-Up Herb Tonic.
3. A stomach-soothing nightcap that works while you sleep, is a tasty way to restore stomach health.
4. Metabolism becomes invigorated through a special herbal combination.
5. Raw juice fast and fruit soup soothe overworked metabolism. For gas relief, stomach cleaning and Super-Plus Stomach Pep-Up, look to folktime healers. Let food be your natural medication!

17

The Natural Way to
Freedom from Aches in the Joints

Phyllis J. experienced a wrenching pain in her lower back when she had to get into her bathtub. She grimaced with a knife-sharp spasm in her midsection when she had to get out of her bathtub. She needed help when getting in and out of an auto. What appeared to be muscular spasms soon resembled severe, shooting arthritic pains. Phyllis J. went the familiar route of liniments and rubs which gave only marginal relief. The pains always came back. She feared becoming a partial invalid, struck down in the prime of her life.

Muscular-Joint Lubrication
Through Secret Greek Stretch

While collecting old books for donation to a local charity, Phyllis came across one volume written by an octogenarian who told of having restored youthful joint-spine lubricity by following an ancient and previously secret Greek stretch-ercise program. He reportedly searched many writings and books until he found this natural, drugless program that was part of the secret of the superior health of the ancient Greeks. It reportedly relieved his joint congestion and helped the body restore its hidden source of *self-lubrication*.

Phyllis J. Unlocks Tight Arthritic Joints

The program was based upon the one followed by the early Greeks. They realized the value of joint health and symmetry.

Stretch-ercise could help the body stir up its built-in source of vital energy, stimulate self-circulation, regenerate the electrolytes to create a feeling of youthful resiliency. Phyllis followed these exercises faithfully even though she experienced a numbing sensation; but after two weeks, she was able to bend over without suffering an agonizing stab of pain in her lower back. By means of the glorious Greek health restoration program of Stretch-ercise, Phyllis J. helped unlock her tight arthritic joints and restore youthful flexibility to her muscular system.

HOW STRETCH-ERCISE HELPS MELT
SORE MUSCLES AND RHEUMATIC SYMPTOMS

This method of organizing the muscles is based on a system of healing taught by the Greeks more than twenty centuries ago. It was one reason for helping this glorious nation reach a peak of physical perfection which is legendary; even today, the beauty of their people is unsurpassed.

Muscle Use Helps Melt Kinks and Soreness

From the age of five, the Greek child began his stretch-ercise education at the *palaestra* (health building gymnasium). He was taught, not muscle development in the usual sense, but the *stretching use* of the muscles. The benefits reportedly were to help melt kinks, soreness, relieve muscular spasms and help put a self-oiling mechanism within the body to work in lubricating the joints and tight parts. Stretch-ercise was beneficial because it helped create an enviable form of perfect coordination and control. Small wonder that they rarely, if ever, suffered from what we today know as arthritis, rheumatism, sore back, muscle aches, stiff back, aching joints and arthritic-like fingers and extremities. They relied upon Nature.

How Stretching Helps Soothe Tired Muscles

The wise Greeks understand the correct relationship of muscular balance. Thus, fatigue was all but abolished to that hardy, healthy and happy nation. The secret here is that you need to establish a "stretching" of certain body parts. This stretch-ercise technique was the secret basis of Greek physical health.

Today, scientists have found that stretching a muscle helps

generate a greater elastic force which produces movement. *Example:* in a steam engine, the elastic force of a gas, generated by fuel-combustion, is converted to energy or "work." This is similar to the process which puts life into the body's tissues, joints and muscular parts.

Stretch-ercise provides a feeling of lightness; almost, a sensation of having conquered the pull of gravity which helps make movements easy and pleasant. The secret here is that the upward stretch of healthful tension is counteractive to the *downward pull of gravity.* It is this downward pull that very often is responsible for arthritic-like symptomatic stiffness.

Progressing Years Signal Need for Stretch-ercise

The ancient Greeks were wise in having the young practice stretch-ercise so as to keep the muscles from stagnating with progressing years. But today, this neglected folk healer is used by a chosen few when they have already experienced the aching symptoms of neglected health. The Greeks realized that with advancing age, the upward thrust of life, which operates in all forms of growth, is the stronger force. After reaching the early middle-years, this "upward thrust" experiences a decline in strength unless the person has learned conservation through stretching.

The Greeks would say that without stretch-ercise, age takes its toll; in their poetic way, they said that it is the same as when the earth begins to reclaim the body. We bend, we shrink measurably, we wither; just as a plant withers and returns to the ground, when the life-force which lifted it and enabled it to withstand the pull of gravity, is used up!

Stretch-ercise Provides Internal Youthfulness

The Greeks maintained that with stretch-ercise, the muscular weight of the body is dispersed along their constantly-moving cords, so that no "dead" weight collects at one point; this means that fatigue poisons do not exert their corrosive action to create stiff soreness and arthritic symptoms.

THE GREEK REJUVENATION SYSTEM OF STRETCH-ERCISE

Here is how the healthy and eternal Greeks were able to produce a condition of "stretch" in every body muscle, including the face for youth, and thus obviate the ravages of arthritic distress:

1. Stand in front of a long mirror, feet together, touching each other. The weight is thrown more forward, on the balls of the feet. The hands are stretched down straight by the sides. Now check your posture. The Greeks sought perfect-posture by being able to draw an invisible line from the ear lobe, through the shoulder, hip-joint and knee, down to the ball of the foot. It is vital to maintain this perfect-posture in order to properly stretch the muscles.

2. Now, draw up from the waist, as if you were trying to pull your upper body (from the trunk up) away from your lower body. Simultaneously, press in your muscles; try to make the front of your waist touch your spine, as it were. This pulling-up action lifts up the rib-cage and the shoulders go along with it. *Caution:* do not raise shoulders separately. Keep them well pressed back. Now, stretch downwards with the thighs and legs, so as to exert as much pull against your upward waist movement as possible. Stretch and counter-stretch; that is the secret as taught in the Greek *palaestra* to the most magnificently healthy people of the world.

3. Next, straighten the neck. Pull it up from the shoulders which are pressed back, you will recall. Extend the neck upwards, as much as comfortably possible.

4. Stretch arms downward, as much as comfortable; push downwards with each finger separately. The arm-stretch creates a counter-stretch against the pull of neck and shoulders. Be careful that the shoulders are not dragged downwards.

5. Against the fulcrum of the stretched and back-pressed neck, push the chin a little forward. Lift it slightly, so that you will feel a pull on the muscles beneath the chin. Now lift the muscles of the face. If difficult, then begin at the chin and smile! The cheek muscles automatically lift with a smile. Slowly, lift the face muscles and the mouth goes with them; hold almost in a pout, until the top lip curves up towards the nose. The cheeks lift until the eyes appear almost half-closed. Now open the eyes to their widest extent. Raise the eyebrows towards the hairline.

6. Finally, brace the muscles of the knee-cap by pushing the knee-cap back as far as possible. Rise up to the ball of the toes. The entire body, from the crown of the head to the tips of the toes, is now in a state of stretch-ercise. Repeat for as long as comfortable.

To Help Ease Stiffness

The facial-stretch may cause a feeling of stiffness that may be uncomfortable. The acid crystals are slowly being flushed out of the veins, capillaries and other body locations and the discomfort may be unusual. To ease stiffness, sit down for the upper body stretch-exercises.

Benefits Require Daily Use

The Greeks maintained that muscles would remain oiled and joints would be youthfully flexible by means of daily stretch-ercising. They require about fifteen minutes at the most and surely are well worth the time when one considers the benefits of joint freedom.

HOW STRETCH-ERCISING CREATES NATURAL FACE-LIFTING

Myra R. used high necklines, intricate necklaces, scarves and mufflers to hide her sagging chin and loose throat. She used various creams and lotions and while self-massage helped provide an emollient reaction and a softening of the skin, there was still the fear of a double or triple chin.

Myra R. learned how stretch-ercise could help firm the stagnant capillaries of the chin when *specifically* applied. When she followed this natural face-lifting program, she was able to pep up her deteriorated chin muscles and the taut muscular pull helped lift up the sag. Now Myra R. need not feel embarrassed about looking older than her husband anymore.

Benefits of Stretch-ercise for Face Lifting

A sagging chin really begins to droop at the waist. It is a culmination of deterioration of posture and slack muscles of the entire torso. The secret of stretch-ercise success in helping to firm up and youthify facial muscles is in helping to "milk" wastes from the muscles of the diaphragm (the muscle sheet that separates the chest cavity from the abdominal cavity). Facial firmness depends upon muscular health generated from the diaphragm; it is the center of gravity from which movement radiates. This following stretch-ercise motion draws from the Greek knowledge of supplying self-washing energy to the region of the diaphragm.

Face-Lifting Through Stretch-ercise

Assume the "top half" stretch position. This time, sit erect in a straight-backed chair. Press the end of the spine against the back of the chair, and draw up the spine as much as you can. Really draw it up, putting energy in the movement.

Try to "pull apart" at the waist, and press in the muscles of the diaphragm and abdomen as hard as is comfortably possible. The shoulders, which are lifted by the stretch-ercise, are pressed well back. Press back the neck. Press the chin a little forward. Lift slightly. Now, raise the muscles of the face and chin. Squeeze up the muscles of the cheeks towards the eyes; squeeze up the eye muscles until they appear as slits. Squeeze as hard as is comfortably possible. Now, against this pressure, try to open the eyes very wide. This Greek-inspired exercise helps firm up face and neck muscles and also helps tone up those related and connected muscles of the waist and diaphragm.

Spine Stretching for Youthful Agility

Health seekers have learned that the spinal column needs to remain flexible, comfortably smooth and rhythmic for freedom from joint aches. Stretch-ercises for the spine help maintain natural lubrication.

The lithe Spanish dancers, Indian women water-carriers and the South American natives have enviable spinal health. They carry heavy earthenware *chatthis* (vessels) of water on their heads, but remain smooth and firm even in advanced age.

The stretch-ercise principle may be taken from the Spanish dancers who perform this rhythm in their art. Their secret of slim, trim waistlines and flat hips? Here it is:

Spine Stretching in Two Minutes Time

Stand up straight. Lift your arms high above your head, trying to reach the ceiling. Pull the body strongly from the waist. Do this as frequently as possible and help lubricate and stretch your spine while youthifying your figure-physique.

HOW STRETCH-ERCISES HELP ERASE WRINKLES

Wrinkles may usually stem from poor circulation. Here are three stretch-ercises used by models and all those concerned about maintaining youth (and . . . who isn't?).

NECK STRETCH   Press fingertips against muscles just below the collarbone and pull downward, at the same time stretching the chin upwards. Move fingertips smoothly, starting at right side and move right over to the left side, holding the upward stretch until you have exercised the entire front neck and chin muscles. Keep your chin pulling upwards the entire time, and you will feel the stretch working the muscles. After each complete stretch-ercise, relax. Repeat up to 10 times.

JAW STRETCH   Make a tight "O" with your lips. Hold this position and roll your lips from side to side.

EYE STRETCH   Squeeze eyes tightly closed. Hold for the count of 10. Open as wide as possible and hold in a fixed stare for the count of 10. Repeat a dozen times or as is comfortable.

When stretch-ercises are followed with a program of health renewal based upon an alliance with Nature through time-tested folklore healers, the rewards may be likened unto the golden keys to a treasure of vibrant youth and health. The ancient Greeks were thousands of years ahead of their time with the secrets of stretch-ercises that help provide juice for the joints!

HIGHLIGHTS OF CHAPTER 17

1. Stretch-ercises are based upon the Greek principle of providing natural lubrication to joints by means of easy stretching.
2. How to unlock tight arthritic joints by means of stretching in simple Greek-inspired motions.
3. Tighten sagging face and chin muscles with stimulating of sluggish muscular cells. Simple stretch-ercises helped Myra look younger than her husband.
4. Spine stretching loosens toxic wastes that may predispose to symptomatic arthritic sore muscular stiffness.
5. How to iron out wrinkles respond with circulation-boosting stretch-ercises.

18

How to Stay Younger and Healthier Through the Natural Power of Autolysis

The natural, self-regeneration process of *autolysis* was well known to the ancients. They would compare the human body to that of a water spring. Periodically, the body becomes steeped with an accumulation of refuse, sludge, impurities, toxic wastes, debris and mucus. Nature causes the spring to undergo a program of *autolysis*, or "self-loosening" and "self-washing" of wastes. Nature provides this self-cleaning of the spring, a systematic breakdown of waste substances through a fermentation process. The refuse-laden spring then becomes sparkling clean through a wondrous cycle of self-purification. The ancients took this secret of autolysis from Nature and applied the same self-cleansing type of process or purification to their bodies.

BENEFITS OF AUTOLYSIS

Regular internal self-cleansing of the body is activated by controlled fasting. Through basic raw juice fasts, special "cellular washing exercises" as well as natural health tonics, autolysis will reportedly perform the following Nature-created benefits:

Clearer Thinking and Mental Magic

Debris-laden blood creates impediments to free blood flow and polluted oxygen to the brain cells. Thought processes need a fresh and clean flow of nutrient rich oxygen available after a self-cleansing program.

Puts Youth-Sparkle into Skin

Autolysis causes a sloughing off of dirt-laden cells and broken metabolic wastes; when passed through the normal eliminative channels, the skin pores become washed. *The skin can breathe freely through autolysis.* It is comparable to the washing of a sieve. The clogged pores now permit normal exhalation of wastes and the skin takes on a youthful quality.

Smooth Hormonal Flow Promotes Vitalic Energy

The endocrine glands issue and promote the flow of the vital life-producing hormones. These glands may be compared to the working parts of any machine or automobile. When they become infested with dirt and grime, they lose efficiency and the machine becomes "old." When the glands are washed and cleansed through autolysis, they can promote a natural life-producing flow of rich hormones and life is youthful and vibrant. No longer is the human machine a tired old wreck.

Improves Nerve Health and
Increases Healthful Functioning of
Your Natural Five Senses

The magnificent nerve network is like any series of wires. It must be kept clean for proper function. Autolysis helps wash away the accumulation of wastes so that the fine wire nerve network need not "twitch" or "jump" at the slightest provocation. In turn, the five senses of sight, hearing, taste, scent, touch, all experience a rejuvenation of power. They become more alert because the nerve system has been "washed" and "scrubbed." Autolysis helps increase the function of these five vital-living senses.

Taps Hidden Source of Muscle Energy

Autolysis helps wash away the accumulation of lactic acid, a fatigue poison that acts as an abrasive corrosion to the muscles and arteries of the body. By washing away other accumulated and related fatigue wastes, the muscles become liberated. Now, the muscle fibers release its hidden source of energy-causing oxygen and glycogen to help the body regenerate itself. Autolysis helps wash away such impurities as carbon dioxide and lactic acid. (Prolonged stagnation may cause an accumulation of lactic acid and wastes that adhere to the end plates or nerve endings of the muscle. Overall body fatigue may occur when lactic acid spills over into the bloodstream.) To tap your built-in supply of energy, wash out accumulated impurities through autolysis.

MORNING SELF-WASHING FRUIT COCKTAIL

Constance R., each morning, takes a special Fruit Cocktail that is all-natural and rich in self-created nutrients that exert an internal self-scrubbing. Constance R. complained of premature tiredness and a feeling of heaviness over her shoulders. In conjunction with Cellular Washing Exercises and one-day-a-week controlled fasting, she has been able to revitalize her system and look younger while feeling younger.

SPECIAL MORNING SELF-WASHING FRUIT COCKTAIL   Each morning, eat a bowl of sun dried apricots which have been soaked in pineapple juice overnight. The secret power here is that overnight, the pineapple juice helps put a dynamic power into the iron and copper of the apricot. The debris-laden bloodstream is washed by the life-giving oxygen that needs extra-powered iron and copper for transportation. This unique, all-natural breakfast helps awaken and revitalize the circulatory system and create a natural self-cleansing. Constance R. finds it is so regenerating, she starts off each day with the cocktail.

CELLULAR WASHING EXERCISES

In a mid-European health center, tired and fatigued patients came for help. While they experienced blessed regeneration through natural foods as well as contrast baths, they needed to free the cemented-like sludge and clogged cellular wastes that festered themselves like mucus to the intricate circulatory channels. Thus was created a set of eight simple exercises that would reportedly help loosen up wastes, remove blockage, free eliminative channels and help cast off these choking sediments.

The principle here is based upon a cup of ordinary tea that has been freshly brewed with leaves. Little sprigs, broken ends of the leaves, minute particles float around in the teacup. The tea is in need of straining and washing, so to speak. This is done by moving a spoon around to catch the particles, to scoop them up from the bottom of the cup, to cast them out. Then the tea is fresh and sparkling and free from hindrance. Too many sprigs create a choked cup.

Cellular Washing Exercises
Loosen Chalky Adhesions

The body's flowing bloodstream is like the tea. The bloodstream often reportedly contains chalky deposits, impurities, deteriorating corrosives that must be sloughed off. Through simple exercises, these chalky adhesions become loosened and then may be freed through normal eliminative channels. The mid-European health center realized that many people dislike exercises so they created this simple set. The benefit here is that each exercise is timed to be exactly six seconds. They require force *without* movement. Here they are:

1. Use a large bath towel for all exercises. Loop the towel behind the neck. Pull your chin in, pull forward on both ends of the towel and resist the towel with the neck, as hard as you can, for just six seconds. Do it only once.

2. Now slide the towel down to the small of your back. While pulling forward on the towel, resist by contracting the muscles in your buttocks and your belly. Push back hard against the towel and count to six.

3. Loop the towel under your left foot and pull up with both hands while your foot pushes down.

4. Do the same exercise under the right foot.

5. Now under both feet, pull up with hands, while your feet push down.

6. Take the towel by the far end, hold towel at thighs and pull hard on both ends of the towel.

7. Now raise the towel high overhead and pull towel hard for six seconds.

8. Now hold towel at shoulder height straight in front of you and pull towel as hard as possible for six seconds.

Cellular Washing Exercises Take Just One Minute

That's right; just one minute helps start the liberation of adhesions and mucus slime that impede normal body functions.

Done regularly, the exercises help start autolysis and self-washing to create life-giving internal cleanliness.

Stiff Bath Brush Awakens Sluggish Circulation

Larry P. was a young 54 and lamented his declining vitality. He felt exhausted by early afternoon; he could no longer keep up with the younger salesmen in his firm and feared loss of his job. The oft-repeated threat of "tired blood" led him to a family friend who told him that the rugged pioneers of the raw and threatening Golden West would revitalize themselves by means of a simple stiff bath brush. It called for scrubbing the body with as comfortable a stiff bath brush as possible.

Larry P. scoffed but secretly tried this plan; he also followed the programs of autolysis that included the Morning Self-Washing Fruit Cocktail and the Cellular Washing Exercises.

Each day, Larry took a lukewarm shower bath. Gradually, he would let the water become cooler and cooler until he conditioned his skin to take it cold. He soaped and washed and then he scrubbed. Oh, how he scrubbed! He used a stiff bath brush and scrubbed his millions of pores until they were as clean as if they had been washed by some magic power. The benefit here is that he scrubbed away the accumulated debris and helped cast off the stored up fatigue-causing lactic acids, carbon dioxide and other chemical abrasives. The pioneers may have derived their stamina from this daily Stiff Bath Brush but as far as Larry was concerned, it was a miracle. Now he took his place with the youngsters and surpassed them in sales.

CONTROLLED JUICE FASTING

The ancients would regularly fast as a means of internal purification. The secret benefit here is that when one fasts, all the body processes are given a rest! This helps strengthen these body processes and give them a refreshed power. Just as you rest your tired feet, so should you rest your internal organs by fasting. The ancients were aware of this natural means of autolysis and their superior intellect, their kinship with God, their amazing powers of vibrant health and cosmic consciousness have remained alive for hundreds of hundreds of centuries. Controlled fasting is an ancient system for washing and resting the internal organs.

Raw Juice Fast

Many prefer a day of raw fruit juice fasting. This helps wash away the accumulated wastes. Others prefer a day of raw vegetable juice fasting. The power of vitamins, minerals, enzymes, amino acids and other valuable detoxifying elements in juices are able to work at self-scrubbing *without* interference of solid food. This may be the secret of autolysis success on a raw juice fast.

One-Day-Per-Week Juice Fast

The ancients would usually fast for one day per week, taking no solids and, often, abstaining from liquids. Today, modern health restoration resorts have found that guests experienced re- markable rejuvenation if they would devote just one day per week to a fast but taking either raw fruit or vegetable juices. This is an easy-to-follow program. *It works while you sleep, too!* Even though *you* are asleep, the nutrients in the juices are awake and working within the system to help scrub away festered mucus and slime. You will awaken with a feeling of restored vitality.

BENEFITS OF FOLLOWING ENTIRE PROGRAM

It is essential for the health seeker to follow the entire pro- gram of autolysis. One grandmother, Edna R., would fast one day a week, but then would stuff herself with heavy sweets, rich carbo- hydrates, stay up late hours, rarely exercise. With such living conditions, autolysis cannot possibly carry out its self-cleansing functions. Edna R. succumbed to arteriosclerosis conditions which required long and expensive hospital and doctor care. She just would not give autolysis its opportunity to self-cleanse her body.

The entire program calls for regular morning exercises, scrub brushing, chemical-free foods, natural foods, lots of rest, controlled fasting. Give autolysis a chance to help you. It costs nothing.

Tub Baths Help Steam Out Toxins

A regular (nightly is preferable) tub bath in comfortably warm water helps steam out the accumulated toxins through the body's pores.

The ancient and healthy Greeks were well ahead of their time in their magnificent baths. Hardly any citizen would let a day go by without a healthful soak. Today, we know that comfortable steaming helps ooze out the festered dirt within our body. Steaming helps to soften and dilute the particles and make them soluble so they can be flushed out through the millions of skin pores.

Most efficient autolysis is favored by a regular comfortable warm steam bath.

HEALTH IS ITS OWN REWARDING BENEFIT

By means of autolysis activity the body takes on the glow of radiant health. Autolysis helps keep the poisons moving out of the body. Self-washing promotes healthful elimination. The eyes are clear, the skin is fresh and youthful-looking, the mouth and tongue are sweet and there is a keen sense of vigorous living. Also, the senses become sharper, the flush of youth creates a feeling of radiant health. Autolysis has helped flush out the retention of toxic material and create a feeling of internal purity that is reflected in lustrous hair, glowing skin, sparkling eyes, limber muscles, flexible joints, lubricated arteries and a feeling of overall youth. *Look to Nature for the secrets of youthful health!*

IN REVIEW OF THIS CHAPTER

1. Autolysis is based upon an ancient method of washing out accumulated wastes and health depleting abrasives.
2. Cellular washing helps improve thinking, youthify skin, normalize a stable hormonal flow, improve nerve health and increase function of the five life-giving senses and promote energy.
3. Morning Self-Washing Fruit Cocktails begin cellular washing program.
4. Just one minute per day for the Cellular Washing Exercises will go a long way in self-cleansing of the body.
5. Controlled raw juice fasts that *work while you sleep* help scrub the insides and promote internal vitality.

19

Folk Healers' Secrets
for Beauty and Daily Good Health

Is it possible to relieve inflammation with a vegetable poultice? Can a headache be relaxed by placing an onion in a certain body part to draw away pain? Will a vegetable help wash out the kidneys? The answer is that these natural folk healers have definitely been promoting health and easing pain for countless previous generations in all parts of the world.

NATURE CREATES HEALING PROCESSES

Throughout the years, my family and friends have been urging me to write down the accumulated folk healers that I have gathered from many little known sources. Some are from old and forgotten books; others are taken from word-of-mouth folklore discoveries. Many come from private sources. They all emphasize natural healing. They are plain. I believe in plain talk. I say quite plainly that these natural healers do not cure you. As you know, even a doctor cannot claim to cure you. He cannot even heal a scratch on your finger—*it is Nature that creates the healing elements that help to induce the body to bring about a healing reaction.*

WHY NATURAL HEALINGS HAVE SURVIVED
THE CENTURIES

Drugs and operative methods on the body have come and gone. Yet natural healings have survived and flourished because of unique benefits their programs impart. Natural healings cause no side effects, are not narcotic, will not become "habit forming," leave no chemical residue in the body system, should not lead to adverse reactions, physically or mentally. Furthermore, they are economical since many of these folk healers are found right in your kitchen pantry or grocer's shelf and cost a fraction of an expensively prepared patent medicine. Nature has created these healers for those who have become discouraged by drugs and pain-killers which reportedly will ease symptoms but provide no cure. For many primitive and modern folks as well, Nature is still the most welcome healer.

Natural Healings Are Easy and Effective

In looking through this book, and specifically this chapter, note that in most cases, natural healings are easy to do while they provide effective comfort. Expect no miracles, though. Not even the so-called "miracle drugs" or "miracle cures" actually live up to their name. But with Nature, there is hope. With Nature, too, there is a need for patience. Give Nature a chance to provoke the dormant healing substances and processes within the body. Now, let us look through the assortment of natural healings:

BURNS AND SCALDS   Following an accidental scalding, folk healers sprinkle icing sugar over the hurt places. Ordinary sugar or even milk is reported to be soothing and helps to heal. If the burn is caused by hot oil or fat, natural healings call for the burned spots to be covered with any type of flour. This helps provide a natural first aid and soothes the fire pain.

SCRATCHES   Folk healers have always used soaked wheat kernels or bran made into a paste with milk. For stubborn scratches, they make a poultice of pulped cabbage leaves (Savoy cabbage is reportedly most effective) and apply to the scratched or wounded region for alleviation. Continue to make repeated cabbage poultices until healing process is effective.

EYE INFLAMMATION OR BURNING   If the eyes have become inflamed through continuous sun or water or snow exposure, folk healers take an egg white, beat it lightly, spread on a cloth and bandage this poultice over the eyes. If possible, they claim, let remain overnight for best results the following morning.

COLD SYMPTOMS   The Romans relied upon the *allium cepa* or the onion to combat cold symptoms. Just cut a slice of fresh, raw onion and immerse it in a glass of hot water. Do not let remain in water longer than two seconds. Sip this water throughout the day. In addition, cut an onion in half and put it on your bedside table; breathe in the smell if you awaken with a stuffed nose. Another folk remedy calls for sniffing a combination of salt water and lemon juice to help unblock stuffed nasal passages.

COLD FEET AND CHILBLAINS   Familiar hot and cold water contrast applications are very soothing. An old folk healer calls for rubbing lemon juice into the feet. Let it dry, then apply olive oil. This provokes a warm stimulation. Cold feet will tingle with pleasant warmth.

TIRED LEGS   Bavarians who climb mountains have reported a rejuvenation of tired legs by soaking the feet in water in which potatoes have been cooked. Afterwards, wrap up in cloths on which you have sprinkled hot, roasted salt. Repeat this procedure until tiredness melts away. The hardy mountain climbers relieve hot, burning feet by the same measure.

PHLEBITIS (Inflammation of the walls of the veins)   An alcohol compress provides primary relief; for added benefit, herbalists suggest the addition of arnica, yarrow or St. John's Wort. After the inflammation has somewhat subsided, apply ordinary clay poultices to be followed by poultices of pulped cabbage leaves. Continue until inflammation is eased.

ABDOMINAL CONGESTION   The time-tested hip bath previously described is often helpful for those who have venous and other congestions in the abdomen.

HEARTBURN   This is often caused by an excess of stomach acid. The simple potato has been used for this complaint for centuries, for relief. Grate one raw potato finely; fold the pulp into a cheesecloth and press out the juice into a glass. Dilute this with twice the amount of warm water and drink regularly first thing in the morning, before lunch and before retiring. It is best to prepare it fresh each time.

GASTRIC ULCERS   Members of the nobility of 18th century Europe often suffered from ulcerous conditions. Court healers would help their overindulgent royalists with a drink made of the juice of a potato and cabbage. It is reported that suffering royalists would drink at least three tablespoons of this infusion before and after each meal with remarkable benefits.

LIVER CLEANSING   If sweet and fatty foods are taking their toll of the liver, then an old healer of cleansing the insides may be helpful. The juice of the common radish has long been hailed by health enthusiasts as a remarkable liver cleanser. Some people add a few tablespoons of carrot juice to create a mineral tonic that is tastefully healthy while it washes the liver, the filtering organ of the body.

GALLBLADDER INFLAMATION   Long before the advent of modern medicine, folk healers would soothe gallbladder inflammation with a compress of cold milk. It was to be renewed every hour until the pain subsided.

DIGESTIVE UPSETS   For overeating, or for distress caused by eating the wrong kind of food, intestinal cramps manifest themselves as digestive upsets. Direct a hot shower upon the stomach. Remain under the shower for fifteen minutes until the skin is flushed. Follow up with a poultice made of raw onion slices.

CONSTIPATION   A time-tested folk healer is that of soaked prunes, taken first thing in the morning and last thing at night. Others have reported relief by taking an herb known as *spring nettles*; this is boiled in milk and taken upon arising.

DIARRHEA   A palatable healer is grated apples. Some prefer raw oatflakes that are to be chewed thoroughly. Nothing else is to be eaten until the diarrhea condition is eased.

HEADACHES   Apply an onion or horseradish poultice to the back of the neck, the soles of the feet. It is claimed many a headache inflammation, such as sinusitis, can be relieved by drawing away the blood from the head through the action of this poultice healing power.

KIDNEY CLEANSING   In the health sanatoriums of Europe, the kidneys receive prime treatment. To help stimulate and strengthen the kidneys, use lots of chopped parsley, preferably raw, in the food or salads. Or, apply a poultice of finely chopped onions to the kidney region to help stimulate their cleansing function.

ITCHING OF THE SKIN (Also known as pruritis.)   This condition is most troublesome and embarrassing. Externally, rub yourself with slices of a raw potato. Or, grate a potato finely and apply the pulp as a poultice.

PIMPLES AND BOILS   Boil ground linseeds (or better still, ground fenugreek seeds) to a porridge-like consistency and apply as a warm poultice to the affected part. Mashed, boiled potatoes offer reported benefits but should be applied as hot as can be borne. This helps "mature" the pus and draw it to the surface. When this is done, cleanse the wound with boiled water. Next, many folk healers sprinkle icing sugar on it and cover with pulped cabbage leaves. Let remain as long as possible.

SWOLLEN FINGER JOINTS   Soak the finger in warm water three times a day, for an hour each time. Take care that the finger is, at all other times, protected from the cold.

INSECT STINGS   If stung by a bee or wasp, the best advice by natural healers is to quickly pull out the sting and forcefully suck out the poison from the affected spot and expectorate it. Resulting pain can be soothed with ordinary garden ivy. Pulp a leaf of this ivy and rub it into the sting. Salt water compresses to which a tincture of ivy has been added is also soothing.

A GATHERING OF BEAUTY-BOOSTERS FROM NATURE

VEGETABLE MASKS   Apply shredded or chopped vegetables of practically all types to the face and let remain until dry. Helps tighten sagging skin and exert a cleansing and tonic benefit.

VEGETABLE OIL   For more of a soft skin, use ordinary vegetable oil to soak into the pores.

EPSOM SALTS   There is something soothing about this ancient and still popular natural healer. Mix a few handfuls of ordinary Epsom salts in a warm tub of water and soak yourself for a half hour. Helps relax and ease congested muscles.

WHIPPED CREAM WRINKLE ERASER   A noted fashion model always depends on a whipped cream facial. Whip up fresh cream, spread over the face. Rub in. Let remain for thirty minutes. Rinse with tepid and then cool and finally icy water. Helps tighten skin and erase the sag that may lead to wrinkle formation.

HAIR HEALTH THROUGH TEA   Before the day of costly (and synthetic) hair shampoos, lovely ladies would use ordinary tea as a hair rinse. The mild acid in the tea would leave the hair in a particularly good glossy condition.

SKIN COCKTAIL   A favorite old-time beauty recipe calls for drinking a cup of hot water with lemon juice before breakfast. Many noted world beauties have been grateful for the action of their favorite skin cocktail.

OIL AWAY SKIN AGING   A complexion beauty secret of many famous beauties is to rub castor oil into the face and neck every day. Let remain as long as possible, then rinse with tepid and cool water. Others have preferred cocoanut or almond oils, which can be bought at a pharmacy, or herbal store.

BEAUTY FORMULA   A famous old-time French beauty, Ninon de l'Enclos, was said to have been a charmer when she was well up into her seventies or eighties. From old diaries, letters and chronicles, we have found that a secret to her ageless beauty may be in this formula: boil one-half pint of fresh milk, one-quarter ounce lemon juice and half an ounce of brandy. While still warm, apply to the face and neck and let dry. This, reportedly, gave the lovely Ninon her ageless beauty.

BUTTERMILK BEAUTY   French Royalists, always aware of the importance of beauty (their lives and their heads often depended upon being beautiful!) would swear by the use of ordinary buttermilk. Not only was it Nature's cleansing drink, but it could be applied to the face, neck, shoulders, arms, etc. It was believed to prevent wrinkles and help stimulate a dazzling youthful skin glow.

WINE WASH   The enviable sparkling youthful appearance of the Spanish was believed to be made possible by this special wine wash. The famed Spanish Duchess of Alba, adored and immortalized by the painter, Goya, as the eternal La Maja, would help keep her skin soft and smooth it is reported, by mixing together half a pint of wine with the juice of a lemon. She would apply this to her face at night. Next morning, she would wash off with warm water. Then she was lovely to look at!

NATURAL HAIR COLORING   For women who wanted to look young and pleasing to the Royalists of Europe, here is a "secret" and natural hair dye. Boil equal parts of vinegar, lemon juice and powdered litharge for thirty minutes over a slow fire in a porcelain-lined kettle. Then comb this mixture through the hair.

HOME BEAUTY TREATMENT   A famed European dancer refuses to let her glorious skin be profaned by chemicals and synthetics. Instead, she follows this home beauty treatment which gives her a youthful look: she begins a bath by first standing in the tub and self-massaging with damp kitchen salt. This creates a natural glow. Then she draws comfortably hot water, adds four tablespoons of olive oil. When she lies down in the tub, she scoops up handfuls of the oil. She massages her body with this oil for fifteen minutes *under the warm water.* She says her smooth, elastic and supple skin is created through this natural home beauty treatment.

HEMORRHOIDS   Commonly known as piles, historical folk healers reported they could be relieved by healing ferns and herbs. They advocate applying a poultice made of *hamamelis virginica* and *calcium fluoratum.* Ordinary cocoa butter is also soothing. Relief is possible by applying a tea made from the tormentilla plant. Also, pulp the spurge plant (regarded toxic if taken internally) and apply as a poultice to the affected region. Many have suggested sponging the region with cold water; this should be done every morning.

NATURAL EYEBATHS   In the case of a blocked tear-duct, a poultice made with horsetail tea will be found to be soothing. Natural eyebaths made of marigold tea or eyebright tea should also be taken advantage of.

CARE OF SUN-TANNED SKIN   Sun-kissed skin is tender skin that requires gentle cleansing. Pure baby soap is the way to cleanse the tanned skin. Lather up the baby soap, gently rub it on with your fingertips and thoroughly rinse away with tepid water. One little cool splash finishes the gentle wash that leaves your tan as soft and glowing as a baby's skin.

HOW TO ACQUIRE A NATURAL TAN   It is reported that you can acquire a base tan slowly by using a mixture of baby oil as a sun screen product on your skin while sunning. Once you have a smooth base tan, deepen and enrich it by using only baby oil. Baby oil contains no sun screen and will attract all of the sun's rays. After sunning, continue oil application to keep your skin lubricated and to prevent moisture loss. The secret here is that natural emollient ingredients in baby oil discourages peeling and flaking and helps prevent dry itchy skin. Lastly, before showering, give yourself a gentle oil rubdown and add some more oil to your bath water to keep your tanned skin baby soft and smooth.

FIVE WAYS TO ANOINT YOURSELF FOR BEAUTY

That pure gentle baby oil your Mom pampered you with when you were little can turn you into a big beautiful baby now. Here are five ways to help stimulate a lovely soft beauty-skin:

1. Before your shower or bath, rub yourself all over with warmed baby oil. It soothes tensed muscles and restores dry skin to baby softness.

2. Soak your hands and feet once a week in a mixture of one-half baby oil and one-half warm water. It gives your feet a soft touch and a soft walk.

3. Treat yourself to a baby oil facial. Warm baby oil and gently massage away old dry surface skin with upward strokes. Rinse with warm water and follow with a cool water splashing. It leaves your skin with the dewy young look.

4. Apply a thin film of refrigerator-chilled baby oil before applying makeup. It prevents moisture from escaping the surface and provides a smooth natural base for makeup.

5. Before going to bed, always remove all traces of makeup (and dirt) with cotton balls saturated with baby oil. Rinse away the stale wastes and then reapply a thin film of baby oil to help protect and regenerate your skin while you sleep.

How to Put a Gleam into Hair   The gleaming crowning glories of Spanish dancers is partly brought about by this ancient secret: Warmed oil is left on the hair for fifteen minutes. Then it is gently steamed out of the hair. The result is lustrous hair.

NATURAL HEALINGS FOR OTHER AILMENTS

Neuritis   It is well known that repeatedly applied compresses of plain hot water soothe pains of neuritis. Still better effects are produced by this healer: soak cloth in melted paraffin. Lay this compress on the inflamed part and fasten with a bandage of wool. This offers partial relief. Take care not to leave the paraffin on too long as you chance burning. A herbal poultice made of slightly warmed St. John's Wort oil is also healing.

Leg Sprains and Ankle Twistings   Many woodsmen of yore would swear by this simple sprain-easing healer. Speed is of the utmost utility in these pain-easing helpers. Take the whites of three to five eggs and beat them until stiff. Add either eucalyptus or camphor leaves (which are good items to have on your herbal shelf) which exert a beneficial strong reaction and help stimulate the blood and lymph circulation which is usually stagnant in sprain areas of the body. Spread the mixture onto a piece of cloth and bind loosely onto the painful body part, using an elastic bandage. The hardening of the egg white should provide a strong dressing. If necessary, renew the dressing in a day's time. Afterwards, massage the affected part with comfrey tincture and also apply cabbage poultices. The woodsmen and simple farm folk maintained that the healing process helped melt pain within a few days.

SPEEDY HEALING FOR SHINGLES (Herpes Zoster)   This disease of the nerves causes "blistering" of the skin in certain areas. This unsightly scaly skin rash remaining after the disease was treated was the plague of folks in past as well as present. Herbal treatments call for a local swabbing solution with extract of lemon balm and marigold.

INSOMNIA   There are many folk suggestions for inducing a sound sleep the natural way. One popular natural sleeping tonic is a tea made of lemon balm (available at most herbalists or pharmacies). A favorite of herbal healers was a mixture of lemon balm, hops and oat juice. Swiss mountain guides know of and use another healer: marmot oil. One teaspoonful of this, taken daily, helped them create a relaxation that induces sleep.

STOMACH ULCERS   Among the many home healers used for stomach ulcers are these: raw potato juice taken regularly; a mixture of raw cabbage and carrot juice. Another medicine from Nature is condensed bilberry and licorice juices (obtainable at a herbalist) taken daily. About 1 to 1½ ounces that are kept in the mouth so that they will become well insalivated (these herbal juices are thick) will help soothe a stomach problem.

ARTHRITIC-LIKE SYMPTOMS   While the folks of the past (and present) century may not have known the technical nature of arthritis, they relied upon Nature for healing. Many expressed relief by applying pulped comfrey roots to the painful parts. Also, tincture of comfrey is soothing as a rub. For added soothing, try butterbur as an herbal rub.

HEALING WITH CLAY

From earliest times, clay has been used to heal many discomforts. Modern beauty specialists rely upon clay for face treatments and outdoor workers know that it will soothe strains and sprains.

How to Make a Clay Poultice   Obtain ordinary clay from a natural health store or herbalist. Mix the clay into a paste and then put on the affected part. Clay poultices may be applied hot or cold, depending upon the individual.

How Clay Soothes Nerves

Take one teaspoonful of clay, add several drops of St. John's Wort oil, mix into a thin paste. Spread this paste about one-fourth inch thick, evenly, onto a piece of cloth and place on the affected part. Let the clay poultice remain overnight to soothe the nerves that are being irritated and cause inflammation.

CHICKEN FAT COOLS SCALDING BURN

Jennifer E. tried to lift a heavy pot with boiling water from the fire. In doing so, she slipped and sustained serious scalding. She might have been scarred had not her husband remembered how his mother would treat all burns and scalds with *uncooked* chicken fat. He spread slivers of uncooked chicken fat over her burned parts. Jennifer felt relieved. She could sleep well that night. Within a week, the pain was gone and in addition to being soothed, new skin began to form. Chicken fat has often been listed as a healer for burns or scaldings.

Some may smile indulgently to read of such simple Nature healers. Let those recall that these healers have been known for hundreds, perhaps thousands of years, and have outlasted many a modern wonder-drug. They are almost always at hand, offer help when there is no help, and we may confidently believe that natural healers will serve the world long after modern drugs and pharmaceuticals have been forgotten and discontinued.

HIGHLIGHTS OF THIS CHAPTER

1. Nature has created a garden of natural healers for common everyday complaints that have been used for hundreds of

centuries throughout the world and are still being used with as good results as ever.

2. Natural healers are beneficial in that they are easy, economical, drug-free, have no side effects.

3. For outer and inner health of your body, natural herbal remedies as recorded from time immemorial are listed in this chapter by type of ailment.

4. The healing ferns, grasses, meadows, trees, and kitchen pantry served our ancestors well in health matters.

20

The Folk Healers' Guide to the Usage of Healing Herbs

The great healing properties of herbs have been recognized and appreciated since time immemorial. With all of our boasted knowledge, we have to admit that our own North American Indian, the primitives of other countries, in their native state, unskilled in letters, with little knowledge of present-day anatomy, physiology or chemistry, were able to prevent and cure with simple herbs those many ailments which still continue to baffle the best efforts of the medical schools.

BIBLE POINTS TO HERBAL HEALINGS

We read in Psalms 104:14 how Moses taught the Israelites to use herbs for the healing of mind and body. The prophet Ezekiel said that the fruit of the tree was for man's meat and the leaves for man's medicine (Ezekiel 47:12). When God created the world and made a beautiful garden, He put the tree of life in it, the leaves of which were for healing. The Lord told them to eat freely of this tree. When man was driven from the Garden of Eden and had no more access to the tree of life, God added herbs to man's diet in the hope it would help heal and contain the human race. The Scripture repeatedly refers to the values of herbs for healing.

Medicinal Properties of Herbs

We know that herbs are able to relieve pain, cause gentle laxative action, stimulate, relieve biliousness, soothe the nervous system, dilute the symptoms of arthritic pain, act as an antiseptic, improve the flavor of foods, soothe inflammation, purify the blood and circulatory system, act as a natural detergent to cleanse the skin, promote an emollient reaction, cleanse the internal organs, relieve various internal and external malfunctionings and also act as a rubifacient (circulation booster) while exerting a natural sedative response. Herbs, more than just healing, are tasty, too! When used in cookery, they improve the healthful flavor of most foods.

Where to Obtain Herbs

Most modern pharmacies and special herbal pharmacies should be able to prepare the desired mixture for you. Many will sell individual herbs. Because herbs come from all parts of the world and may be sold in certain localized areas, it is prudent to ask the pharmacist to obtain herbs that he may not have in stock. Inquire at health stores. Look in the classified telephone directory of any large city under Herbs for possible mail order service.

HOW TO GATHER YOUR OWN HERBS

It should be understood that wide experience and knowledge of herbs is needed to successfully gather and preserve these healing grasses. Soil knowledge is also necessary. Plants grown in natural, organic and virgin soil will contain far greater healing value than those grown on poor soil. The same herbal plant grown in different localities will show a great variation in the amount of healing properties they will yield. There is also a difference between cultivated plants and those growing in their natural wild state. For example, the dandelion growing wild has amazing medicinal properties which are almost entirely lost when the plant is cultivated. Wild herbs are more effective for healing use than those grown in the garden.

When to Gather Herbs

Horticulturalists suggest gathering herbs only in dry weather, preferably when the plant is in full bloom, or the seeds getting ripe.

BARKS   The barks should be taken when the sap is rising in the Spring. Shave off the outer rough part, then peel the inner part from the trunk of the tree. To dry, put in the sun for a short time (if desired), then complete the drying in the shade. Be sure they are thoroughly dry. If there is any moisture left in them when they are put away, they will mold.

ROOTS   Dig up the roots either in the Spring when the sap is rising, or in the late Autumn, after the sap has gone down. Slice and dry the roots (in the shade), tie up in small bundles and put in the attic or some place where they are sure to be kept dry.

FLOWERS, SEEDS, LEAVES   Gather when they are in their prime and gather only the perfect ones. These should also be dried in the shade. When thoroughly dry, put in heavy brown paper bags.

STORAGE   Do not preserve herbs in glass, as sometimes the glass sweats, and if any moisture comes in contact with the herbs, they will become moldy. When any barks, roots or other herbs are thoroughly dried and kept dry, they will retain their potent value for years.

DRYING TIME   The barks, roots, flowers, seeds or leaves may all be dried for a short time in the sun, but always complete the drying process in the shade, as too much exposure to the sun tends to reduce the healing value. They may be dried entirely in the shade in an airy place. The only thing gained by putting them in the sun for a short time is hastening the drying process.

HOW TO USE HEALING HERBS

GRANULATED OR FINELY CUT HERBS   Steep a heaping teaspoonful of the herbs in a cup of boiling water for twenty minutes, strain and take one cup an hour before each meal and one cup upon retiring. You may take more or less as the situation warrants. If too strong, use less herbs per cup.

ROOTS AND BARKS   Roots must be simmered thirty minutes or more in order to extract their medicinal value. Do not boil hard. (When you gather your own roots and barks, cut or crush them fine. If you raise or gather herbs and barks, use good judgment in making teas; if you get it too strong, add more water.)

FLOWERS AND LEAVES   These should never be boiled. Steep them in boiling water in a covered dish for twenty minutes, just as you would make common tea. Boiling evaporates the aromatic properties.

POWDERED HERBS   These may be mixed in hot or cold water. Use one-half teaspoon to one-fourth glass of water. Follow by drinking one glass of water, either hot or cold. The herbs reportedly take effect quicker if taken in hot water.

Sensitive Stomach

Those who have sensitive or abused stomachs may become nauseated after taking some of the best old-fashioned herbs. In such cases, start by taking teaspoonful doses of herbal tea, often—about every fifteen minutes—and increase the amount as the stomach regains its health.

Herbs in Foods

Powdered herbs may be mixed with foodstuffs such as mashed potatoes, mashed vegetables of any kind, sweet fruits like dates or figs, also ground into food. You may add a little honey to herb tea, to make it more palatable.

How to Make Herb Salves   Use fresh leaves, flowers, roots, barks or the dried granulated or powdered herbs. (If you gather the herbs yourself and use them fresh, be sure to cut up finely.) Use one pound of herbs to 1½ pounds of any pure vegetable oil and four ounces beeswax. It is necessary to use a little more beeswax in the warmer climates as this is the ingredient that keeps the salve firm. Mix the above together, cover, and place in the hot sun or oven, with the fire turned low, for three or four hours. Strain through a fine sieve or cloth. When cold, it will be firm and ready for use. It can be used, however, before it is cold.

Herb Poultices   To make any of the following poultices, it is best to have the herbs in a ground or granulated form. When using the herbs ground, mix with just enough water to make a thick paste. When using the herbs granulated, mix with water, cornmeal or flaxseed meal to make a thick paste. If fresh green leaves are used, beat them up, steep and apply to the affected parts.

What Herbal Poultices Can Do for Your Health

Herbal poultices reportedly soothe enlargements such as eruptions, boils, abscesses. For benefits-plus, first bathe the affected part thoroughly with mugwort tea, before applying the poultice. In applying poultices, the purpose is to retain warmth and moisture as long as possible. Renew sufficiently to prevent cooling or becoming dry.

How Herbal Liniments Promote Healing

For most blemishes, pains, bruises, boils, the ancients and moderns, too, relied upon herbal liniments. Many have found relief from headaches by applying herbal liniments to the temples, back of the neck and forehead. *To Make Herbal Liniment:* combine two ounces powdered myrrh, one ounce powdered golden seal, one-half ounce cayenne pepper, one quart rubbing alcohol (70%). Mix together and let stand seven days. Shake well every day. Then bottle in a corked bottle. Rub into affected region periodically and let dry in.

HERBAL NERVE-RELAXANT   This reportedly has many healing qualities that will soothe, relax and quiet the nerves. Combine equal parts gentian root, scullcap herb, burnet root, wood betony and spearmint herb. Then mix one half teaspoonful in one glass cold water; follow with a glass of piping but comfortably hot water. Take one hour before each meal and one hour before retiring. Helps create a pleasant sleeping disposition.

HERBS FOR FEVER-COOLING   In conditions of fevers and colds, herbs have been found to create a cooling reaction. A favored herbal powder is made of these healing grasses: 4 ounces bayberry, 2 ounces ginger, 1 ounce white pine, 1 dram cloves, 1 dram cayenne. (Use all powdered herbs.) Mix and put through a fine sieve twice. Steep one teaspoonful in a cup of boiling water about fifteen minutes, covered. Drink the clear liquid poured off from the sediment.

YOUR HERBAL HEALING GUIDE
AS REPORTED BY ANCIENT WRITINGS

Based upon ancient, forgotten Nature-cure books, scrolls, parchments, writings, here is a treasure of herbal healers that offered life to those who looked to the woods and forests for natural tonics.

Acidosis

Golden seal, taken one-fourth teaspoon in a glass of hot or cold water an hour before meals, is beneficial. Other reported herbs are burnet, sanicle, wood betony, calamus, peppermint.

Asthmatic Allergies

A suggested tonic herb: equal parts of lobelia, wild cherry bark, scullcap, gentian valerian, calamus and cubeb berries. Mix thoroughly and use a heaping teaspoonful to a cup of boiling water. Drink one cupful of this herbal tonic three or four times a day and one cupful upon retiring. If you do not have all these herbs, use two, three or more that you have.

Catarrh

In this condition, there is an excess of waste accumulation. To improve breathing, a nasal wash consists of a pint of lukewarm water and one teaspoonful of salt. Repeat until breathing is comfortable. An herbal gargle is made of the following: one teaspoon of powdered golden seal to one pint of boiling water. Let it steep for a few minutes and then pour the liquid carefully off. Add one-half teaspoon boric acid and snuff it up the nose and then gargle with the same solution. This reportedly is cleansing, soothing and healing.

Circulation Tonic

Any of these herbs, made into a tea, help pep up a sluggish circulation: gentian root, scullcap, colombo, rue, valerian, vervain, peppermint, spearmint.

Constipation

If possible, take an enema made of the juice of red raspberry leaves, wild cherry bark or leaves or bayberry bark, using one heaping teaspoon to a quart of water. This reportedly is a good stimulant as well as a cleanser. One suggested HERBAL LAXATIVE: mix thoroughly one tablespoon each of mandrake, buckthorn bark, rhubarb root, fennel seed, calamus root and one teaspoon of aloes. If powdered, take one-fourth teaspoon in a half glass of cold water, followed by a glass of hot water. May be taken after meals or upon retiring. Take more or less than the one-fourth teaspoon, according to severity of constipation. EXTRA-STRENGTH HERBAL LAXATIVE: Mix thoroughly one ounce mandrake root, one ounce cascara sagrada bark, one ounce buckthorn bark, one ounce fennel seed, one ounce calamus root, one-fourth ounce aloes. Put through a fine sieve to mix thoroughly. Take one-fourth teaspoon with a glass of hot water upon retiring.

Colitis

Use a teaspoon of golden seal and one-fourth teaspoon of myrrh to a pint of boiling water. Let it steep. Take one tablespoon of this herbal tonic six to eight times a day. For severe cases, take one tablespoon every hour.

Dyspepsia (Sour Stomach)

Golden seal, taken one-quarter of a teaspoon to a glass of water an hour before meals, will offer relief. Or steep one teaspoon in a pint of boiling water. Drink one half cup an hour before meals. Healing herbal teas made of scullcap or gentian, taken every three hours, will be soothing. Other reportedly soothing herbal teas may be made from the following natural healers, either singly or in combinations of two or three: tansy, wild cherry, magnolia, sweet flag, masterwort, golden thread, gentian root, boneset, buckbean, horehound, quassia, spearmint, wahoo, thyme, summer savory, yarrow, white oak, peach leaves, myrrh.

Dropsy

This usually refers to an accumulation of watery fluid in the cellular tissues or in any of the other body parts such as the legs, chest, arms, etc. The ancients brought welcome relief by means of inducing a natural perspiration; they would drink plenty of red raspberry tea (made from dried raspberries). Another herbal healing tea that was used is made from equal parts of: wild carrot (blossoms or seeds ground), dandelion root, yarrow, burdock, queen of the meadow, dwarf elder. Then use one teaspoon to a cup of boiling water and steep twenty minutes.

Eczema

For skin tone-up, herbs offer hope. Take equal parts burdock root, yellow dock, yarrow and marshmallow (the herb, not the synthetic food). Use one heaping teaspoon of this mixture of granulated herbs to one cup of boiling water. Steep, strain and drink one-half cupful some five times a day. Also soothing is to bathe the affected skin parts freely with this same tea.

Ear Trouble

Home remedies usually call for the application of soothing heat over the ear and around the neck. Another folk healer is to bake a large onion until it becomes soft; tie over the ear to provide relief when pain is severe. A poultice may be made of lobelia or slippery elm. Also, a saturate solution of boric acid may be used for a wash.

Fevers

Old-timers always helped break up cases of fever with such herb teas as made from red raspberry leaves or willow bark or, especially, slippery elm. This last herb is regarded soothing to the stomach and intestinal tract, also has a powerful self-cleansing action. Folk healers use any of these herbs made into a tea and sipped until the fever abates: yarrow, red sage, peppermint, wild cherry bark, valerian, black cohosh, tansy, camomile, elder, bone-set, willow (bark or leaves), marigold, nettle and lobelia.

Felons

This is the old name for a modern condition we know as a painful abscess, usually on the end of a finger, thumb or toe. It may be caused by a blow or injury when the skin tissues become bruised. An old healer is to insert the finger or toe into a hollowed out lemon and let remain there for a long period of time as possible or convenient. An excellent poultice is made of equal parts of slippery elm, lady's slipper and lobelia herb. Granulated herbs can be used if powdered is unavailable.

Gallstones

In the days before doctors were available, known gallstones were said to respond to several herbal and natural healers. A hot fomentation of lobelia and hops over the region of the liver was said to sooth distress. Hot herbal teas that would ease gallbladder upset are made of: equal parts of as many of these herbs as can be obtained: hyssop, gentian root, nerve root, scullcap, buckthorn bark. Mix thoroughly and use one heaping teaspoon to a cup of boiling water. Take one cup of this herbal tea every hour, the first day. Then continue to take four times a day, one cup an hour before each meal and upon retiring. This reportedly will help liquefy the bile and improve liver health.

FOMENTATION for Gallstones: This was used to ease gall-stone problems before modern medicine. A half hour after taking the herbal tea, follow by taking four ounces of olive oil and four ounces of lemon or grapefruit juice, beaten thoroughly together. After taking, lie on the right side with the hips elevated by placing two pillows beneath them. This causes the oil-juice mixture to run along the region of the gall bladder, creating a natural lubrication. Fomentations of lobelia and hops will reportedly provide soothing relief to the pain and also help improve lubrication of the gall bladder duct to permit oiling by the lemon juice-oil mixture. GALLBLADDER RELIEF THROUGH HERBAL TEAS: one rounded teaspoon of powdered wood betony, or one of milkweed mixed in one-half glass of cold water; follow by drinking a glass of hot water. Take one hour before each meal and upon retiring.

LEMON JUICE-OLIVE OIL TONIC   Take two tablespoons lemon juice, followed by two tablespoons olive oil, or vice versa, on an empty stomach.

Gout

This is a form of arthritis that is known to respond to proper diet. Herbs often reportedly provided healing benefits. Herbalists would suggest: take equal parts of scullcap, yarrow, and valerian, granulated. Mix thoroughly together and use a heaping teaspoon to a cup of boiling water. Steep and drink one cupful an hour before meals and one upon retiring.

HERBAL TEAS   Any of the following are soothing. They may be taken singly or in any desired combination. Use a total of one teaspoon to a cup of boiling water; steep twenty minutes and drink four cups a day, an hour before each meal and one upon retiring. Herbs for gout include: blue violet, burdock, gentian root, mugwort, rue, birch, broom, sarsaparilla, buckthorn, ginger, pennyroyal, plantian, wood betony and balm of Gilead.

Stomach Gas

Peppermint and spearmint tea help relieve accumulation of fermented gas. Equal parts of calamus root, valerian, with granu-lated peppermint should be mixed together; use one teaspoon to a cup of boiling water. Steep, strain and drink one half cup an hour before meals and another half cup after meals.

HERB STOMACH STRENGTHENER   To create a self-cleansing of gas, take one fourth teaspoon powdered golden seal in one half glass of warm water an hour before meals.

Coughs and Respiratory Congestions

Hot herb tea made of sage or red sage is soothing. Hyssop, yarrow, black cohosh, peppermint and camomile teas also healers. Take several cups throughout day.

Chronic Bronchitis Conditions

Take equal parts of wild cherry, mullein, coltsfoot, yarrow, horehound and buckthorn. Mix together, using one teaspoon to a cup of boiling water. Take one cup four times a day.

HISTORICAL HERBAL TEAS   These were used in pre-modern medical days for those who looked to medicines from the meadows for healing of bronchitis—chickweed, coltsfoot, cubeb berries, golden seal, lungwort, mullein, myrrh, white pine, sanicle, saw palmetto berries, slippery elm, white pond lily, yerba santa, bloodroot, ginger, blue violet, bethroot, red root, red sage and lobelia. For a tea, use singly or in desired combination.

Burns and Blisters

Herbs were used to heal burns. Take one teaspoon of golden seal, one of myrrh and one of boric acid and add to a pint of boiling water. Let the mixture stand 30 minutes; then pour off the clear liquid and apply with absorbent cotton. This reportedly exerts a healing reaction. For a deep burn, healing is facilitated by sprinkling on the sore in dry form, using just the powdered myrrh, golden seal and boric acid.

HERB TEA   This was said to help stimulate circulation and improve healing possibilities—take one teaspoon each of valerian, scullcap and peppermint. Mix together and use one teaspoon to a cup of boiling water. It is said to be quieting and soothing to the nerves which usually are more frazzled than the burn!

Bed Sores and Chafing

Hot and cold applications and thorough rubbings help bring about a good circulation. A healthy wash is made of witch hazel and water applied to affected regions. Another good wash is made of one teaspoon each of golden seal, myrrh and boric acid to a pint of boiling water. When the sore has been washed, it should be sprinkled with equal parts of dry golden seal and myrrh. This helps allay the infection and offers a healing relaxation. Cover with a little cotton or oiled cloth.

Headaches

Relief is often possible by taking a hot foot bath to which has been added one tablespoon of mustard. Herbal teas may be made of peppermint, valerian, spearmint, black cohosh or scullcap. For relief before retiring, take one cupful of hot hops tea. One reported herb tea is made of red sage, said to be one of the best for headache relief.

Hiccough

This is usually due to the irritation of the phrenic nerve which causes contractions of the diaphragm. One traditional treatment is the old-fashioned one of eating a slice of lemon with a few drops of Angostura bitters on it. A stubborn case may respond to onion juice in teaspoonful doses. A poultice of one-half teaspoon cayenne pepper to a pint of vinegar thickened with cornmeal, whole wheat flour or linseed meal, applied to the diaphragm, is reportedly helpful. A herbal tea made of blue cohosh, black cohosh, taken separately or mixed, equal parts, is soothing.

Hemorrhoids

A natural herbal suppository is made of the following: 2 ounces powdered hemlock bark, 1 ounce golden seal, 1 ounce powdered wheat flour, 1 ounce boric acid, 1 ounce bayberry bark. Mix with glycerine, then apply to the affected region in the form of a suppository.

Nervous Conditions

For those who are nervous, who are given to fits of anxiety, sudden fear, indigestion, temper, Nature offers hope. Suitable nerve-soothing herbs are: black cohosh, blue cohosh, valerian, vervain, skullcap. Use a heaping teaspoon of any of these herbs to one cup of boiling water. Drink one cup every three hours. It is also soothing as a Herbal Nightcap to take one cup before retiring.

Herbal Hair Massage

Ancients suggested taking the leaves and bark of the willow tree; make into a tea and apply to the scalp to help conditions of dandruff and falling hair. Any one of the following herbs were used to nourish and brighten the hair of the ancients before synthetic chemicalized tonics came on the scene: nettle, pepper grass, sage, henna leaves, burdock. Steep a tablespoon of either of these herbs in a pint of boiling water for 30 minutes. Then add one level tablespoon boric acid. Massage the scalp with this solution. Rinse in tepid and then cold water.

Itching

Wash the affected part with tar soap. Then take one tablespoon of each of these herbs: burdock root, yellow dock root and yarrow. Steep in a pint of boiling water for 30 minutes. Strain, put in a cooking pan (do not use aluminum), add one pound of vegetable fat or vegetable oil. Boil slowly, stirring frequently until it has boiled down to the consistency of salve. Apply as any salve and use as a healing lotion. It is reportedly beneficial for most ordinary cases of skin itching and eczema.

Bladder Distress

When too much starch or sugar is ingested, there is distress that often manifests itself as bladder upset. The herbal healers would put faith in this natural laxative: equal parts of senna, buckthorn bark, spearmint, cubeb berriers and marshmallow. Mix together. Take one teaspoonful to a cup of boiling water. Drink up to four cups a day. For soothing bladder: take one heaping teaspoon of golden seal in a cup of piping hot water.

Jaundice

When the natural healers saw a yellowish skin, they recognized it to be caused by bile obstruction. Other noted symptoms included yellowing of the whites of the eyes, a bitter taste in the mouth, constipation, dark urine, slight fever, headache and dizziness. The herbalists suggested taking one-fourth teaspoon golden seal in a glass of water, one hour before meals, three times a day. A raw fruit juice fast was reportedly helpful in restoring an acid-alkaline balance and also to wash out the toxic wastes. Herb teas made of (singly or in combination) dandelion, yarrow and agrimony were said to be good.

FOLK HEALER   Grandma would take a handful of peach pits, grind or crush them. She would make a tea by putting them in two cups of water and letting them simmer for 30 minutes. She would take one-fourth cup of this tea upon arising every morning, the same amount before each meal and at bedtime.

Night Sweats

The time-tested home healer is to take a hot salt water sponge before retiring. Use two tablespoons of salt to a quart of water, or a hot bath followed by a salt glow. A soothing tea is made of one tablespoon golden seal steeped in a pint of boiling water and sipped before retiring.

Prostate Disorders

Even before folks knew the name of this problem, they looked to the ferns, grasses and roots of Nature for healing. They would rely upon a poultice of slippery elm applied to the crotch. A soothing tea is made of equal parts of gravel root and leaves or peach leaves. Use in combination or singly and drink when thirsty throughout the day.

Arthritis Disorders

While there are many forms of rheumatic-arthritic disorders, the natural healers recognized that herbs could provide a feeling of flexibility to stiff and aching joints. In conjunction with corrective diet and exercises and the programs outlined in this book, herbal teas have reportedly been helpful to sooth arthritic-like symptoms. Mix equal parts of these herbs: black cohosh, gentian root, angelica, columbo, scullcap, valerian, rue and buckthorn bark. Use one heaping teaspoon to a cup of boiling water. Steep and drink frequently throughout the day.

HERBAL POULTICE   Two tablespoons mullein, three tablespoons granulated slippery elm bark, one tablespoon lobelia, a small teaspoon cayenne. Mix thoroughly together. Mix with enough boiling water to make a stiff paste spread on a cloth (about one-fourth inch thick) and cover the swollen joints with this poultice. Replace when needed. PAIN-RELIEVING POULTICE: equal parts of oil of origanum, oil of lobelia; add a few drops of oil of capsicum. Apply full strength (or mix with cocoanut oil) and massage as a natural liniment upon aching parts.

Sinus Distress

Old-time healers would use contrast applications over the region of the sinuses to help unblock congestion. A herbal inhaler is made as follows: make a tea of bayberry bark by using one teaspoon to a cup of boiling water. Let it simmer for 30 minutes. Strain. When comfortably cool, sniff it up the nose, getting it up both sides, one side at a time. This helps create a gentle freeing of congestion.

Sore Mouth

For conditions of mouth cankers or sores, it is best to abstain from acids and drink much vegetable juices. A good *herbal mouth wash* is made as follows: One teaspoon golden seal, one-half teaspoon myrrh, steep in a pint of boiling water. Add one tablespoon boric acid. When settled, pour off clear liquid. Use as a mouth wash leaves in a cup of boiling water. Strain through a cloth. Saturate or a gargle, as desired. Also, white oak bark, wild alum root, red raspberry leaf tea used as a mouth wash or gargle is soothing and naturally healthful.

Eyewashes

Because the eyes are delicate, it is wise to use natural healing and herbal based washes. For those who worked by candlelight or kerosene lamps, an eyewash refresher was made as follows: steep one teaspoon of red respberry leaves, one teaspoon witch hazel a soft cloth with this herbal wash and apply as a wet pack to the eyes; or, just bathe the eyes with it. Fennel tea, diluted one-third with water, was also a traditional eyewash for those who labored under poor lighting conditions. For eye inflammation, charcoal or slippery elm poultices applied cool to the eyes were reportedly soothing.

FARM FOLKS EYEWASH   Take one teaspoon golden seal, one level teaspoon boric acid, dissolve in a pint of boiling water. Shake well. Let settle. You may pour off the liquid or use just as is.

How Herbs Help Stomach Health

For a "happy stomach," look to the woods and the treasures of the forests. Reportedly, red raspberry tea is soothing to the stomach. Many abstain from plain water and drink tea made from red clover blossoms and/or leaves throughout the day. Other good "happy stomach" teas are made from either of these herbs: sage, wood betony, poplar bark, bitterroot, slippery elm, colombo, hyssop, plantain, wild yam, sweet flag, yarrow, strawberry leaves, wild alum root, rue, violet leaves. STOMACH BALM: mix equal parts of golden seal, echinacea, burnet, wood betony, myrrh, and spearmint (use powdered herbs). Mix thoroughly together and take one-half teaspoon in a glass of hot water about an hour before each meal and then before retiring.

Wounds and Cuts

Before the availability of chemicalized patent medicines, wounds and cuts were treated with herbal kindness for healing. Here are some suggestions drawn from folk healing sources. Tie a bandage on the cut immediately to stop the bleeding. You may wash the cut or wound with a solution of powdered golden seal and myrrh. Steep a heaping teaspoon of each in a pint of boiling water for twenty minutes. Provides a natural antiseptic benefit. If the cut bleeds freely, tie it up in its own blood; this helps it heal readily. *For a large cut:* place it in the golden seal and myrrh solution, as hot as can be comfortably borne. Continue this, keeping the solution hot until the wound closes. When it is almost closed, press it together, sprinkle a little powdered golden seal on the outside and then bandage.

POULTICES   Wood sage, self-heal, chickweed, golden seal, myrrh, slippery elm, are medicines from the meadows that can be used as poultices and washes for cuts and wounds and skin blemishes.

Coughs and Sore Throats

A cough may be interpreted as Nature's symptom that the body system must be cleansed. Most patent medicines contain narcotics, addictives, drugs and chemicals that reportedly cause side effects, repress the cough yet do not exert any restoration of health that will eliminate the condition responsible. Let us dip back into the healing lore of the past and see what herbalists would use for conditions of coughs and sore throats.

COUGH SYRUP   Take one teaspoon each of colt's foot, black cohosh, cubeb berries. Mix thoroughly and steep in a pint of boiling water. Take a glassful every hour.

SWEET COUGH SYRUP   Boil a quantity of strained honey or malt sugar and add to the cough syrup to give it a sweeter taste as may be desired. The rich supply of potassium in honey is also soothing to the throat.

HERBAL BERRY TONIC   Steep one teaspoon of cubeb berries and one-half teaspoon lobelia in a pint of boiling water. Drink when comfortably warm. This helps cut the phlegm, cleanse the throat and stomach of toxic mucus.

HERB TEA FOR THROAT-EASE   One teaspoonful of strong pennyroyal tea taken every 30 minutes is soothing. Make this tea by using a heaping teaspoon of the granulated herbs (or one-half teaspoon of the powdered herb) to one cup of boiled water. Sweeten with honey, if desired.

HERBS FOR HEALING THROAT DISTRESS   Make a tea of any of one or two of the following herbs and drink three cups a day, an hour before meals. Tansy, wild cherry bark, hyssop, mullein, flaxseed, horehound, pepper weed, cubeb berries, white pine, spikenard, colt's foot, blue violet, palmetto berries, thyme, golden seal, red clover blossoms and lobelia.

*   *   *

We have not come so far from the days of natural healing. Today, a rich treasure of folklore healing is waiting to be discovered. "Speak to the earth, and it shall teach thee," says the Good Book (Job 12:8). We may well draw upon the hundreds of centuries of healing secrets for today's "wonder" cures. Healing is brought about by the restoration of the entire person. Just as there is no singular cause of illness, so there is no singular treatment. Ally yourself with Nature and her ways of working with your body and reap the rich rewards of God-endowed health.

Index